Praise for the Transplant Tetralogy series

"His wit and style are as compelling as his tightly wound thriller plots, and his thoughts on the world we live in are fascinating and, often, spot on... An awe-inspiring feat."
Washington Post

"Fitzhugh's stuff is unique. It's also alarmingly accurate. That's what makes it so good." *Clarion-Ledger*

"Bill Fitzhugh just gets better and better." *Christopher Moore*

"A thrilling tale of science run amok... laugh-out-loud send-ups of the madness of modern life." *Booklist*

"Fast, funny, deft action... You have to experience it, hanging on tight and keeping those pages turning."
New Orleans Times-Picayune

"Where Bill Fitzhugh earned his Ph.D. in street smarts is a mystery. The wicked sense of humor he must have been born with." *Dallas Morning News*

"Genuinely funny... his satiric eye spares no one."
Publishers Weekly

T0174414

A Perfect
HARVEST

THE TRANSPLANT TETRALOGY, BOOK 4

BILL FITZHUGH

This edition published in 2021 by Farrago,
an imprint of Duckworth Books Ltd
1 Golden Court, Richmond, TW9 1EU, United Kingdom

www.farragobooks.com

Print ISBN: 9781788423304
Ebook ISBN: 9781788423298

Cover design and illustration: Christopher Sergio

1

My name is Leonard Stratton and I'm going to tell you a story. The story is true and it's tragic, though it's not without its own dark humor. So if you feel the urge to laugh somewhere along the way, by all means, indulge yourself. But this is a story I promised to tell and, being a man of my word, tell it I will.

It is a story about the young man who died saving my life and the lives of many others, though they are not the ones whose lives he set out to save. In fact none of these people should have been in danger in the first place, yet they were. And before it's all over, you will see who was to blame for that, something you will find deeply satisfying if, like me, you're the sort of person who believes it is always important to assign blame.

The young man's name was Miguel Padilla, may his soul rest in peace.

Since, as they say, you can't run the experiment twice, there is no way to know for a fact but I believe this story would not have happened the way it did without Miguel's two best friends, one of whom is a lawyer, the other a doctor. The lawyer's name is Kristine Black. The doctor is Javeed Ahmadi.

Miguel, Kristine, and Javeed met as undergraduates at UCLA and became fast friends, "the three inseparables" if I might borrow from Dumas' *Les Trois Mousquetaires*. This would make me d'Artagnan, a character I have seen described as a young, handsome, brave, and clever man. Though, to state the obvious, I'm not as young as I once was.

In any event, and without getting into how good I look for my age, or so I'm told, here's what happened…

***

On Friday, November 6, 2015, Miguel drove to the Los Angeles Medical Complex where his friend, Dr. Javeed Ahmadi, an internist with an excellent reputation, kept his office.

Miguel spent the day undergoing a battery of tests, traipsing from room to room, machine to machine, in one of those breezy gowns with his chestnut-brown cheeks playing peek-a-boo every other step. And you can imagine a few of the nurses sneaking a peek as Miguel was, in fact, a handsome man in good shape. At least outwardly.

A quick bit of background: Miguel and Javeed were from different neighborhoods in the San Fernando Valley in greater Los Angeles. Miguel's family traced to somewhere south of the border but how far south, I have no idea. Javeed's family, as you may have guessed from his name, came from somewhere in the Middle East. More specific I can't tell you. Persian or Arab? I don't even know the difference and in the end it doesn't matter.

In any event, late of the afternoon in question, after the tests, Javeed was back in his office waiting for Miguel. On the walls of his office hung a collection of diplomas and certificates. On his desk were plastic anatomical models of the heart, brain, and kidney. In one corner of the room, displayed on a rolling stand, was a full-scale replica of a human skeleton. A plastic version, mind you. The real ones cost around six thousand dollars and what's the point in spending that sort of money when you can get a perfectly good model for a hundred bucks? Especially if you're not in orthopedics.

Javeed was pouring over the test results when Miguel came into the office and took a seat. Javeed looked up from the file and said, "You want me to beat around the bush for a few minutes or dive right in?"

"Just go for it," Miguel said.

"OK," Javeed said. "You have amyotrophic lateral sclerosis. ALS. It's a progressive neurodegenerative disease that—"

"Lou Gehrig's disease?"

"I'm afraid so, Miguel. I'm very sorry."

Miguel had only the vaguest sense of what this diagnosis entailed except that it was a slow death sentence. "But that's... that's, uh..."

"Terminal and incurable? Yes it is." Javeed said this more casually than he intended.

Miguel gave him a look of disbelief. "I was going to say 'that's not good.'"

"Oh, sorry. You're right, it's not good. Not good at all."

"Wow." Miguel stood and began to wander around the office in a daze. "I, uh, wasn't really prepared for that. I mean, we knew something was wrong but... How long do I have?"

"It's hard to say."

"Do your best for an old pal, would you?"

"Three to five years is average," Javeed said. "Some live ten years or more. But there *are* outliers."

"Yeah, anyone I'd know?"

"Well, for example, Stephen Hawking. He lived till he was seventy-six, I think, so..."

Miguel seized on this thin bit of hope. "Seventy-six? So, that's good news, right?"

Javeed shook his head. "Not really," he said. "Toward the end, the man only had a single cheek muscle that still worked. So it depends where you land on the quality of life question."

"Damn. So, what happens?"

"Muscle weakness starts in your hands and feet. You'll start to drop things and you'll stumble. Later it affects your speech, swallowing, and breathing. The usual cause of death is respiratory failure. Essentially you'll suffocate."

"Are there any treatments? Anything to slow it down?"

"Miguel, I'm not going to lie to you." Javeed gestured out the window at the Medical Complex and said, "There's plenty of snake oil out there, but nothing I'd hang my hopes on."

"Again, wow. OK. Well, I appreciate you being honest with me." Miguel stared out the window but at nothing in particular. "So that's it? It's all over? Three years or so and I'll be dead?"

Javeed rubbed at the back of his neck and looked somewhat chagrined when he said, "Yeah, listen, Miguel, it gets worse."

Miguel turned to look at his friend. "How can it get worse? You just said I'm going to die."

Javeed picked up a folder. "I know. I'm so sorry but you remember the tests we did?"

"Yeah, I'm pretty sure I was there when we did them."

"Right, well, we found something."

"You just said, Lou Gehrig's Disease."

"Yeah, well, we found something else with the MRIs." Javeed pulled a scan from the folder and showed it to Miguel.

"OK, so what am I looking at?"

"It's a glioblastoma, I'm afraid."

"That doesn't sound good."

"Oh, it's definitely not," Javeed said. "It's a brain tumor. Highly malignant and growing like... hell, I don't know, growing like a family of rogue Mormons."

"Joseph H. Smith! A brain tumor? Are you serious?"

Javeed nodded gravely. "Afraid so."

"So that might explain the periodic spasm of blinding pain in the center of my head?"

"Yeah, most likely."

"Alright, in this race to kill me, who's going to win, Lou Gehrig or the brain tumor."

"The good money's on the glioblastoma."

"In other words, the good news is I'm not going to die from Lou Gehrig's disease."

"Most likely not."

"So, this brain tumor. Is there some way to treat it?"

"I'm afraid so," Javeed said. "And, to be completely honest, it's horrifying. Worse than the cancer if you ask me."

"Javeed, would it kill you to soften this up the tiniest bit? You know, show some compassion or something?"

"Miguel, I know you. You don't want any bullshit, right?"

"True enough, but…"

"This? What I'm giving you? It's the truth," Javeed said. "It's ugly and I'm sorry, but I figured you'd want it straight."

"I appreciate that, but you know what they say about a spoonful of sugar helping the medicine go down? Couldn't you sweeten this up at least a little?"

"Sure, in Mary Poppins' world, that's true. But they didn't have glioblastomas at Number 17 Cherry Tree Lane and I don't want you to have any illusions about what you're facing."

"Well, mission accomplished." Miguel stood in front of Javeed's wall of diplomas, considering the news. "Jesus, so what am I looking at? And you're right, no bullshit. Give it to me straight."

"OK," Javeed said. "There's nothing to be done about the ALS. But if you want to give it the old college try with the tumor, you should know it starts with a craniotomy, by which I mean they saw off the top of your skull and try to remove the octopus-like tendrils of the tumor, but they won't be able to get it all so after they scrape around a bit they'll slap the top of your skull back on like a bony beanie cap before putting you through a hellish round of chemo and radiation, the side effects of which will make you wish you were already dead." Javeed took a sad, deep breath before saying, "And then you'll die."

"Well, at least you weren't callous about it." Miguel picked up the plastic model brain from Javeed's desk and looked at it, trying to imagine the octopus-armed glioblastoma spreading over his cortex. As he rotated the model in his hand, it slipped, breaking into its instructive pieces on the floor. He looked up at Javeed.

"That's how it starts, the neuromuscular part. You lose control."

Miguel was on his knees picking up the pieces when he had what he believed was a revelation. "Wait a second! Hang on! How common is this?"

"Is what?"

"Lou Gehrig's disease. How many people get it every year?"

Javeed gave it a moment's thought. "In the U.S.? Something like two in every hundred thousand, so it's rare."

Miguel put the pieces of the brain back on Javeed's desk. "And what about this alleged brain tumor?"

"The glioblastoma? About the same rate, so, again, pretty rare."

"You took statistics, right? So answer me this: if the odds of getting either one of these is that rare, what are the odds I'd get both?"

Javeed could see where this was going, but played along. He said, "The odds are absolutely astronomical, Miguel. No question. It's like winning the lottery but with fewer tax implications."

"Exactly! Don't you see? The test results got mixed up."

"You're suggesting my diagnosis is wrong?"

"No offense intended."

Javeed waved it off. "None taken. Let me show you something." He pulled the MRI scan from the folder and pointed at it. "See that? That is a classic glioblastoma. That image is so perfect it is going to be in a tumor textbook some day." He slipped the scan back into the folder. "I'm sorry, Miguel, but there's nothing faulty about the diagnosis."

"You've obviously got someone else's MRI."

"Ohhh. And the ALS?"

"You got the wrong chart or you misinterpreted the data, or, no wait! I've probably got something that mimics the ALS."

"Miguel, I agree that would be possible if we hadn't ruled out peripheral neuropathy and myopathy with the electromyography and the nerve conduction study or the infectious diseases like HIV, human T-cell leukemia, polio, and some others that cause ALS-like symptoms."

"Fine, but, the point is, it doesn't matter *how* it happened. The point is the odds on this must be a trillion-to-one. There's just no way…"

"Ironic, isn't it?"

"What?"

"This." Javeed gestured at Miguel. "What's happening right now."

"What's happening?"

"My friend, the psychology teacher, doesn't recognize that he's in denial about this."

He struggled to keep from saying, "I am not!" Instead he looked at Javeed who offered a kind smile. "OK, maybe I am. A little."

"It's understandable, Miguel." Javeed started across the room to offer some comfort to his friend. "You just got some awful, life-changing news." Javeed spread his arms to give Miguel a hug. But instead, Miguel took a swing at him. Javeed dodged the punch and, strictly out of instinct, slugged Miguel in the stomach, doubling him over and dropping him to one knee.

When Miguel got his breath back, he looked up at Javeed and said, "Jesus! Why'd you hit me?"

Javeed thought that was pretty rich, so he pointed out that Miguel had thrown the first punch.

"I mean, why would you hit a dying man?"

"Trust me," Javeed said. "That's not what's going to kill you. Anyway, this is good!"

"It's good that my dear friend and my doctor is gut-punching his dying patient? How is that good?"

"It means you've moved from the denial stage to anger. That's progress. And quick." Javeed helped Miguel to his feet.

"You'd be angry too," Miguel said. "I don't deserve this. I haven't really lived yet. I thought I had more time. I mean, I've been putting things off and working hard so I could get the joy out of life, you know… later."

Javeed gave a sage nod and said, "Well, if you haven't made a bucket list yet, now would be a great time to start."

Miguel seemed to surprise himself when he said, "I have no idea what I'd put on it."

"OK, all right, let's think." Javeed paced a bit, snapping his fingers before he said, "Have you tried… I don't know… heroin? Or sex with a man? Or—"

"What?"

In that moment an ambiguous look crossed Miguel's face prompting Javeed to ask, "Wait, are you considering the smack or the sex?" He quickly waved his hands, erasing the question. "Never mind. I don't want to know. I'm just saying, the constraints are off! You're free to do whatever you want! It's a dream come true!"

"For fuck's sake, Javeed, I'm dying!"

"I know, but you got, like, a two-minute warning. Most people don't get that. You've got time to have some serious fun without worrying about the consequences."

"So I should just descend into… debauchery?"

"Just think of the possibilities!"

"No! I'm not just giving up. There's got to be something I can do to fix this."

Javeed felt the best thing to do at this stage was to play along, so he said, "Oh, OK. Let's try bargaining. Have you considered prayer?"

"I'm agnostic, for god's sake. I need to do something real and concrete. Something practical." He turned and wagged a finger at Javeed. "In fact, the first thing I need is a second opinion."

"I thought I *was* your second opinion."

"OK, a third and a fourth opinion. I need to find a doctor who knows what the hell he, or she, is talking about."

"And I encourage you to do that. You're bound to find a quack out there somewhere who'll tell you everything's gonna be alright."

"And I'm going to look into alternative therapies!"

"There's this woman in Santa Monica who swears she can heal just about anything with her healing crystals."

"Not that kind of thing! Real therapies. I bet they're doing stuff in Europe and Asia we can't do here either because of regulations or the medical-industrial complex can't profit from them."

"You might want to give Laetrile a shot."

"And I'll change my diet! Start eating kale and quinoa."

"Be sure to add some essential oils."

"Mock me all you want, but I bet diet's a big part of it. I've heard stories about people with multiple sclerosis who switched to a Paleo diet, next thing you know they're running marathons!"

"Ah." Javeed stared at Miguel for a moment before he said, "So not just alternative therapies, you're also going with alternative facts?"

Miguel didn't seem to hear what Javeed said. He found himself looking at the skeleton on the rolling stand. "Oh, who am I kidding? I'm going the way of all flesh." He took its bony hand and said, "Just like you. So let me ask, what happens when you die? Do you lose all your fears and regrets?"

"He wouldn't know. He's plastic."

Miguel looked the skeleton straight in the eye sockets. "What was it the poet said? Do not go gentle into that good night, old age should burn and rave at close of day, I think. But I'm not old. I'm just… dying. And there's nothing I can do about it."

Miguel grasped the pole that supported the skeleton and slid slowly down to the floor as all hope slipped away. "It's hopeless," he said. "It's all over. I'm going to be put to bed with a shovel." He was quite melodramatic.

Javeed couldn't help it, rolling his eyes at Miguel's theatrics. "Would you stop that?"

"I've wasted my life. And now what? I just wait for the suffering? The morphine? The numbing 'til death arrives?" Miguel looked up at the window and began to crawl toward it. "Maybe I should just end it myself."

Javeed made a point of checking his watch as he said, "Are you done yet? It's past five."

Miguel glanced up, irritated at his friend. "This is the depression stage!"

"No shit, I get it. But if you would just get to acceptance…" Miguel reached the window and tried to get it open. "What are you doing?"

"I'm going to jump! Save myself the suffering."

"Hate to break it to you, Miguel, but the window doesn't open. Even if it did, we're on the second floor. You'd just break an ankle or something. Come on now, get up, brush yourself off and we'll go somewhere and talk about your alternatives."

"I've got alternatives?"

"Sure, like gin or vodka for starters. Come on, I'll call Kristine. She'll want to be there for you." Javeed helped Miguel to his feet.

"I guess you're right. So, I'm going to die. It's not going to be today and, besides, no one gets out alive, right? I can't take it too seriously."

"Exactly. You need to take a minute and step back to think about things. You need some perspective."

"Actually, what I need is a drink."

2

Before we get to the bar, I should warn you that many people are going to die before this story is over. Most of the dead won't literally be *in* the story and if that confuses you at the moment, don't worry, it will become clear in time.

One of the deaths will be a murder. Or maybe it's a suicide—it's an odd death. No, actually, the death itself isn't odd. Death is death, after all, merely the cessation of life. It's not as though a man pulled the frozen head of a swordfish from the freezer and stabbed someone through the heart. *That* would be odd. It's more a matter of perspective on who caused the death and, I suppose, the question of murder or suicide is debatable in this case, more so than in the old law school brainteaser about the guy who… Well, I'll let Kristine tell that one since she's the lawyer. She will join us in a just a moment. In any event, here's what happened next.

Miguel and Javeed went to a place near Javeed's office on the southern edge of the Medical Complex, a restaurant and bar called The ICU, as in Intensive Care Unit. The place featured waitresses in skimpy nurse outfits and bartenders dressed like surgeons, serving drinks in specimen jars, that sort of thing. It was popular with the hospital crowd and medical fetishists.

They were at a table near the back working on their second round of drinks. They were drinking bourbon, but there was a martini glass and a shaker on the table waiting for Kristine.

Javeed was looking at his phone, reading from a web page as he said, "But keep in mind that from that height, you hit the water at seventy-five miles an hour. Your spine snaps, your liver splits, ribs break. It might not even kill you, though you're likely to drown before help arrives."

Miguel peered over the rim of his glass. "OK, let's scratch that one."

"Fine. How about the Second Amendment approach?" Javeed made a gun from his fingers and put it to his head.

Miguel shook his head. "I don't own a gun. Plus, it's too messy." He looked into his glass, swirling the whiskey. "Hey, what about pills and booze? I've always liked the sound of that."

Javeed scrolled through the page before he found the facts. "I'll be damned, pills and booze only works about two percent of the time. I wonder why." He scrolled up. "Oh, here's a classic. Carbon monoxide poisoning."

"The old car in the garage trick?"

"Yep. Nice and peaceful, no mess, and a higher success rate than pills."

"That would be perfect except I own a Prius."

"Fine, you can die from being smug."

"Is that it?"

"No, there's plenty more," Javeed said. "How about the old head in the oven?"

"Again, mine's electric."

"You're not making this easy, are you?" Javeed glanced up and saw Kristine making her way through the crowded bar as fast as she could. "She's here."

She arrived, arms outstretched. "Oh my god, Miguel, I'm so sorry, I can't believe it! I don't know what to say." She wrapped her arms around him and held on for dear life.

"You don't have to say anything. I'm just glad you're here."

Kristine broke their embrace and wiped the tears from her eyes before pointing at the martini on the table. "Is that for me?" She sat down and gulped it.

"We figured you might want one," Javeed said, pouring her another from the shaker.

Kristine put her hand on Miguel's. "How do you feel? I mean, are you… in pain or anything?"

"No, I'm OK for now, thanks."

Kristine held up her glass and said, "Miguel, may every hair on your head turn into a candle to light your way to heaven and may God and his holy Mother take the harm of the years away from you."

Javeed raised his glass and said, "Salud!"

Miguel shook his head and touched his glass to Kristine's. "Thank you for your beautiful toast." They took a drink then both gave Javeed a disapproving look.

"What?" Still holding his glass in the air.

Miguel said, "Salud means 'health,' you stupid camel jockey."

"No way. It just means, 'cheers,' right?"

"I'm pretty sure I've got this one since it's Spanish," Miguel said.

"My mistake," Javeed said, hoisting his glass again. "Here's to my friend, the wetback know-it-all." The others joined the toast and ordered another round.

Miguel looked at Kristine and said, "Listen, after the news, I started thinking. I haven't done my will or anything and, time running short and all, I was hoping you could handle that for me."

"Sure, of course. Will, trust, powers of attorney, advance directive, whatever you need." She held up her phone. "We can open a file now if you want."

"There's an app for that?"

"Of course." Kristine opened a form on her phone and filled in the blanks. Miguel Padilla. Single. No children. Parents deceased. No siblings. "You have any relatives I should know about?"

"Nothing but distant cousins."

"Alright, let's talk assets."

Javeed leaned in to say, "He's got a Prius and an electric oven, but he doesn't own a gun."

"I've got some equity in my house, some retirement savings, some small investments, that's about it." Hearing the words gave him pause. "So not much really, when you stop to think about it. Not much at all."

"OK, where do want your estate to go? Who inherits?"

"This is new territory for me. I've never really thought about it," Miguel said. "I'll get back to you on that."

"Not a problem," Kristine said. "When do you need this?"

"There's no hurry," Javeed said. "He's dying, but he's not setting any world records."

"Javeed!"

"It's true," Miguel said. "And Doctor Feelgood here says it's going to be a miserable death when it comes, which is why we're discussing potential suicide methods."

Kristine looked at Javeed with disbelief. "You didn't tell him about AB-15?"

"I was about to! I wanted him to get it out of his system first."

"What's AB-15?"

"The End of Life Option Act the governor just signed. Physician-assisted suicide in case you want to skip all the unnecessary suffering."

Miguel turned to glare at Javeed, who responded, "I said you had alternatives!"

"You said gin or vodka. Remind me again why I don't consider you a complete douchenozzle."

"Because you know I love you, we're best friends, and because of our whole fraternity thing."

The three of them lifted their glasses to toast, proclaiming as one, "*Lex clavatoris designati rescindenda est!*" They laughed and downed their drinks.

Kristine poured a third martini from the shaker before leaning over to hug Miguel. "This is so unfair! I don't want you to die!"

"I'm not crazy about the idea myself, but what are you gonna do?"

"You know we're here for you. Whatever we can do, just name it."

"Fine. For starters tell me about this AB-15."

"It's pretty simple. You get two doctors to confirm a diagnosis of terminal illness that will, within reasonable medical judgment, lead to death within six months. You also need to be mentally competent for making and communicating your healthcare decisions. After that you go home with a big dose of… something." She looked at Javeed.

"It's either Seconal or Nembutal, I forget which. But either way, you get nine or ten grams of that in your system and your troubles are over. So not bad, right? I mean, it beats the alternatives. That's why I was saving it for last."

"You're a prince," Miguel said.

"You think you want to go that route?"

"Can you say with any 'reasonable medical judgment' that I've only got six months to live?"

"Not really. I suspect you've got a little more than that," Javeed said. "But I think you'll want to get the ball rolling as soon as possible, in case you decide you want to do it. I suspect the bureaucracy for something like this is a nightmare."

"And you can always decide not to do it," Kristine added. "Even after you've submitted paperwork."

Miguel nodded his understanding.

"So," Javeed said, "you want me to start the paperwork on that?"

***

That's the sort of question that will make you stop and think.

I mean it's one thing if you're at a dinner party and the conversation takes a turn in that direction and someone asks if you would, theoretically, under some distant, alien circumstance, want your doctor to start the paperwork on your means of suicide immediately after a terminal diagnosis, right? You'd sip your drink and say of course. Or maybe you would say of course not, you preferred a painful death. I suppose some people are bent that way. But it's something else entirely when your actual doctor asks if you're ready to place that to-go order for death-with-dignity and it's no longer a theoretical matter because it's actually staring you in the face.

And the question gave Miguel pause. But not for the reason he would have guessed.

Of course, like a lot of people, Miguel had thought about end-of-life decisions before now. But, like a lot of people, that thinking had been done from a safe distance. From the vantage point of youth and health, as part of a thought experiment in college, or following a grandparent's funeral or a news story about a young person suffering from some horrid, disfiguring, and painful disorder.

But now, here it was, nothing theoretical about it.

Miguel had always come down on the self-determination side of the equation, the one espousing that at some point in the life cycle, the individual's right of autonomy surpassed whatever the state's interests were in denying that right. That was still his position and firmly held at that. The problem now was that the question had actually been posed. It was no longer academic. So it wasn't just a matter of taking a position on the issue. Now it was a matter of taking action based on that position.

So, he wondered, how do I answer?

And for the moment at least, Miguel's answer still counted. He still had decisional capacity. But for how long? He knew he would lose it at some point. This was another reason to get Kristine working on the legal documents. The advance directive. The POLST. The power of attorney for healthcare. Because without those… Miguel knew it was the lack of expressed pre-commitment that had caused so much trouble for Karen Ann Quinlan, Terry Schiavo, their families, and so many others over the years.

Miguel thought he might also write a letter of intent. Short, sweet, and unambiguous. Pull the plug. Do not intubate. Do not resuscitate. No nasogastric feeding tube. No respirator. None of it. Let me go and say goodbye. Miguel wanted to make damn sure he wasn't left to wither into the fetal position, ending his life like a sixty-two pound piece of dried fruit.

***

"Miguel?" Javeed said. "You want me to start the paperwork?"

Miguel said, "No."

"No?"

"No."

"Why not?"

"I can't. Not yet anyway. Weren't you listening just now? I've got nothing to show for myself."

Javeed said, "Your Prius is in pretty good shape."

"You know what I mean," Miguel said. "I haven't done anything with my life."

"Well, not to put too fine a point on it," Javeed said, tapping the face of his watch, "but you better hurry."

"You're not kidding. I don't have time now, do I? Not to do anything significant, anyway. I mean, it's not like I've got time to find the cure for brain tumors, though wouldn't that be great?"

"Yeah, but you'd still have Lou Gehrig's disease, so..."

Miguel flipped Javeed off and continued, "Seriously, I have nothing of consequence to leave behind. I have no... legacy, nothing to show that I was here, that I made a difference in the life of a single person."

"Miguel, that's not true!" Kristine took his hand. "You've done a lot of great stuff. You've volunteered services, you've donated to charity. And think of all the students you've touched over the years."

The phrase hung in the air as Miguel looked at her.

"Whose *lives* you've touched. You know what I mean."

"This is more depressing than the diagnosis." Miguel sounded demoralized. "I just wish there was something I could do to show that I was here, that I cared, that I made a difference in this world."

There was a long pause as Miguel considered his uninspiring existence. Javeed spent the time looking into his glass. Kristine glanced toward the ceiling until she said, "Oh! What if you could… no, never mind. That won't work."

Another moment passed before Miguel said, "Hey, how about if I started a… no, that's not gonna happen."

Again, they paused in search of an answer. The silence was broken when Javeed slapped a hand on the table and said, "Wait wait wait wait just a minute." He hesitated as he checked for flaws in his plan. "No. I've got it!"

"I'm listening."

Javeed delivered this with the same confidence as he had Miguel's diagnosis. "You, my dear friend, can make an enormous difference in someone's life and the lives of that person's family and friends. You can do something truly remarkable, extraordinary, something heroic!"

"That's fantastic," Miguel said. "But hurry up, would you? My doctor tells me I'll be dead soon."

"And right he is," Javeed said. "But in the meanwhile, you can give… the gift of life!"

Miguel was confused. The gift of life? "What, like knock somebody up? Leave a fatherless child behind?" He glanced at Kristine.

"Don't look at me. I'm not raising a kid on my own, even for this project."

"No! You can save someone's life!"

"How?"

"You can donate a kidney to someone."

Miguel's eyes brightened for the first time that day. "Well that *would* be something, wouldn't it?"

"They've erected statues for people who have done less," Kristine said. "That's a great idea!"

"It's brilliant," Miguel said. "But can I donate with the cancer and everything?"

"Sure, brain transplants aren't a thing and, for now, the rest of your organs are fine," Javeed said. "You just can't wait too long."

Miguel leaned across the table, took Javeed's face in his hands, and kissed him on the forehead. "This is fantastic! You're a genius!"

"I knew you would realize that eventually. Thank you."

"So what do we do?"

"We just find someone who needs a kidney, which is pretty easy since there are about twenty thousand people in California looking for one. You can donate to a relative, a friend, or a complete stranger as long as you've got a tissue match. But either way, you save a life."

As Javeed explained the advantages of a live donor kidney versus a cadaver kidney, Kristine was on her phone doing some research into the matter.

"Javeed's right," she said. "I don't see anything here that disqualifies you from being a legal living donor. And here's something interesting. This is from the National Kidney Foundation website. It says living donors can also donate parts of their lung, liver, and pancreas."

"That's true, I hadn't even thought of that," Javeed said.

"So I could save three or four people? *That* would be remarkable!"

"That would be legendary!" Kristine said.

"But…" Miguel's mind raced toward the logical extension of the conversation.

"But what?"

"But why stop there?"

Javeed looked confused. "I don't follow."

"Why stop with saving three or four people? Why not donate everything?"

"Well because… what do you mean, everything?"

"Just what I said. Kidneys, lungs, liver, pancreas, heart, whatever anyone needs."

Javeed shook his head. "You can't do that until you've been declared brain-dead."

"How come?"

"That's just the legal protocol."

"OK." Miguel turned to Kristine. "How do we get around that?"

"Not my area of the law, but it's an interesting question."

"Just so I'm clear," Javeed said. "You want to know how we can render you brain-dead so we can harvest all of your organs?"

"That's not exactly what I'm asking, but please, if you have an idea…"

"The only way I'm familiar with is the method the Chinese are famous for using," Javeed said. "But you're not going to like it."

"Try me."

"They figured out where to shoot their political prisoners so they were brain-dead but not dead-dead. Then they could keep them on a vent until they had buyers for all the organs."

"Great," Miguel said. "So all we need is a member of the People's Republic of China's firing squad."

"And a gun, since you don't have one."

"Seriously, why can't they just put me under and take my organs?"

"Well it's technically feasible but no surgeon would ever do it."

"Why, because of the whole, 'first, do no harm' thing?"

Javeed shook his head. "You know, those words aren't actually in the Hippocratic Oath."

"Really?"

"Yeah it's sort of implied, but that's not a quote. I don't know why people keep saying it. But to answer your question, a surgeon wouldn't do it because it would be considered homicide."

"Oh." Miguel frowned and said, "I can see how that would get in the way. But what if I agreed to it?"

Kristine said, "You can't agree to be killed. U.S. law doesn't recognize the concept of consensual homicide."

Miguel pointed at Javeed. "What about you? You'd do it for me, right?"

"What? You want *me* to kill you?"

"What're we friends for?"

"I'm serious," Javeed said. "You're asking me to ruin my career! To go to prison. I can't believe you would put me in the position to have to answer that just to make up for your lack of accomplishment in life."

"That's a bit harsh, don't you think? But you're right," Miguel said. "That's too much to ask. I'm sorry I went there."

"It's not that I don't *want* to kill you," Javeed said.

"So we're back to one kidney and portions of my lung, liver, and intestine."

"Pancreas."

"Whatever. What's a pancreas even do?"

"All sorts of stuff," Javeed said. "It's endocrine function is to release enzymes into the small intestine for digestion. It also has an exocrine function and it makes insulin. It's a dandy little gland."

"And just think of the impact you would have on the people waiting for those transplants," Kristine said. "Think of their spouses, their parents, children, friends. That would be so great!"

"It's good," Miguel said. "But I think we can do better."

"How?"

"I don't know. I just have the feeling we're on the right path but we're stopping before we get to the end of it," Miguel said. "And I think this is the thing I need to make me feel like I've accomplished something with my life. Let's get back to AB-15 for a second. So the state has passed this law that gives me the right to die, but only in the way they prescribe."

"Yeah, so?"

"So right now, if I had an accident or a run-in with someone from a Chinese firing squad and was rendered brain-dead, I could donate all of my organs?"

"Yes."

"How many organs can you donate?

Javeed said, "A perfect harvest? Eight."

"In other words," Miguel said, "if we do the living donor thing and stop at four, we're leaving some perfectly good organs on the table."

"Another way to look at that," Kristine said, "is you're also putting some perfectly good people in the morgue."

"Out of curiosity," Miguel said, "how many people are waiting for transplants?"

"In the U.S., somewhere north of a hundred thousand last I heard," Javeed said. "About twenty-two people die every day on the waiting lists."

"Can I donate my organs if I go the AB-15 route?"

"Afraid not. That's done at home and by the time they get your carcass to the O.R., your organs wouldn't be viable. It has to do with the period of detrimental warm ischemia relative to allograft function, which is probably more than you want to know, so…"

They ordered another round of drinks and sat in thoughtful silence for a moment. Kristine thinking about how much she would miss Miguel when he was gone. Javeed trying to conjure a medical miracle for his friend. Miguel inadvertently eavesdropping on the people at the next table, just soaking up all the humanity around him while he still could.

He heard one of the men talk about how important this one thing was to him now and both of the women confirmed his observation before going into careful details about how best to do the thing he wanted. And they all were deadly serious about it.

After listening for a minute Miguel said, "One good thing I can think of in light of the fact that I'm dying is that I will no longer have to worry about shit like whether I'm moisturizing enough."

"What? You've been worried about skincare?"

"It's crossed my mind," Miguel said. "I mean, nobody wants to be ashy, but so what? Slap on some lotion and move on. Don't get paralyzed worrying about whether your exfoliating regimen is sufficient or whether you need to take it to the next level?"

"There's a next level?"

"That's what I hear," Miguel said, nodding at the adjoining table. "And all this time I've been all calm, cool, and collected about my skin situation when it turns out I should have been in a black panic about not having a go-to hydrator. Can you believe it? I've been carrying on, casual-as-you-please, when I should have been focused on whether using serum on top of a moisturizer is going to ruin my hydration game. I didn't even know I was supposed to have a hydration game! So imagine what a relief it is to realize how many more stupid things I no longer have to worry about."

Kristine wasn't surprised to hear Miguel didn't have a go-to hydrator. She had noticed some dry skin issues but didn't think it was her place to call him ashy and she was about to comment on that when she noticed the bartender carding a twenty-something across the room and a thought occurred to her. She held her hand out to Miguel and said, "Give me your wallet."

He handed it over saying, "There's no moisturizer in there if that's what you're looking for."

She pulled his driver's license. "What's this?"

"My driver's license."

She pointed at something on the license. "This."

"Oh, that's the little organ donor sticker," he said.

"That's right," she said. "According to the California State Department of Motor Vehicles, you are an organ donor."

Miguel took his wallet back and pulled a card from inside. "I also have this." He handed it to Kristine.

"Well, well, well. A state-issued organ donor card," she said. "The plot thickens."

Javeed drained his drink and said, "How so?"

"Because Miguel has made two legally binding declarations that he desires to be an organ donor, something he has a lawfully guaranteed right to do free from interference." Kristine did a Google search on something.

Javeed said, "But with AB-15, the state is…"

23

"…interfering with that right," Miguel said.

Kristine read from her phone, "A properly signed declaration is a legal document under the Uniform Anatomic Gift Act and is effective to authorize donation in every state."

"OK, so?"

"So with AB-15 the state has given its approval for you to end your life," Javeed said. "But only by their approved method."

"But their approved method prevents you from donating your organs," Kristine said. "Catch-22."

"What's worse, it ensures eight other people will die," Miguel said. "I'm no lawyer, but that's… depraved indifference or reckless endangerment or something. It's got to be something to let eight people die who don't have to, right?"

Javeed said, "So you're accusing the state of what? Conspiracy to commit murder?"

"I'm not sure what it is," Miguel said, "but I don't think any of it's kosher."

Kristine slapped a hand on the table. "I think you have a solid equal protection argument."

Javeed replied, "OK, so?"

"So we're going to sue the bastards!"

3

On Saturday morning, Miguel and a slightly hungover Javeed Ahmadi were in Miguel's living room waiting for Kristine so they could begin work on their historic legal challenge.

"So let me ask you this," Javeed said, as he sprawled on the sofa, one arm draped over his bloodshot eyes. "Why do you think the church made suicide a mortal sin?"

"Because they found it immoral?"

"Don't be naïve," Javeed said. "They did it for the money."

"The money? What money?"

"You can't tithe if you're six feet under, right? But if you're threatened with mortal sin and eternal damnation, you might keep yourself above ground and putting money in the plate."

"I'm going to take your word for it."

"Sure," Javeed said. "And the government made suicide a crime for the same reason the church made it a sin. Dead men don't pay taxes."

"Is any of that true?"

"No idea," Javeed said. "But it sure has the ring of truth, doesn't it?"

Miguel glanced up at the clock in the kitchen. "You told her nine o'clock, right?"

"Yeah, and here's something to think about while we wait. Back in the day, when there *were* laws against suicide, you know what they actually criminalized? It wasn't *whether* you killed yourself, it was how quickly you did it."

"You're going to have to explain that."

"OK," Javeed said. "Back then, if a young man took the easy way out, the authorities would go after his estate. If he tried and failed? They'd throw him in prison. But if he killed himself slowly with booze and cigarettes and working in the coal mine for a decade, they didn't give him a second thought when he croaked. You know why? Because by then, they'd already gotten their money's worth out of him."

Miguel was about to ask a follow-up question when the doorbell rang. He answered it, letting Kristine in. "You're late," he said. "Where've you been?"

"Thinking things over," she said.

"Great, what's the plan?"

"You're not going to like it."

"How come?"

Kristine looked Miguel in the eyes and said, "Miguel, I hate to say this but I think we should forget the whole thing."

"What?"

"I know. But in my professional opinion, it's a bad use of your time and your money."

"OK, but it's my time and my money, so I say we go to court."

"I'm just being realistic," she said, glancing toward the counter separating the kitchen from the living room. "Thank god, coffee." Kristine went to the counter and poured a cup.

Miguel followed. "What the hell happened? Last night you were ready to take the case to the Supreme Court!"

"That was the alcohol talking," Kristine said, slightly embarrassed. "You had, what, two martinis?"

"I had three," Kristine said. "And if I'd had a fourth, I'd have been willing to go *down* on the Supreme Court. You know I don't hold my liquor very well. I say forget the lawsuit. Instead, donate one of your kidneys while you still can and let that be your legacy. That would be huge!"

"What? No!" Miguel was shocked by the betrayal. "Absolutely not. I'm not surrendering my rights without a fight!"

"Miguel, lawsuits are expensive, they're lengthy, and the results are unpredictable. And that's before the appeals start," Kristine said. "Trust me, you'll be dead long before the case ends and all you will have donated is your money to some lawyer."

"That's why we file an emergency petition seeking immediate declaratory relief!"

"Oh Christ." Kristine rolled her eyes. "One year of law school and you're Clarence Fucking Darrow."

"Hey, I aced Civil Procedure!"

"And then you dropped out and got your Master's in Psychology whereas I graduated law school, passed the bar, and… point is, we'll never see the inside of a courtroom."

The truth, or what Miguel believed to be the truth, suddenly dawned on him. "Ohhh. Now I get what you're saying."

"I knew you would," Kristine said. "I just don't think we can win the case, certainly not in your lifetime. And if not, what's the point? Donate a kidney and call it a day."

"No, you're saying you don't think we can win… with you as counsel."

Javeed smirked at this from the safety of the sofa.

"What? No, this isn't about me," Kristine said. "It's about the way the system works."

"You're afraid you can't win the case."

"Miguel, you know how slow the courts are. You said it yourself, you aced Civil Procedure."

"That's right, and then I dropped out and got a Master's in Psychology. You know the law, I know people. You're afraid you'll lose."

"You don't know what you're talking about."

27

"So what was it, a traumatic experience in moot court? My guess is you lost real bad to a rival in front of your favorite professor."

Kristine stared at Miguel for a moment before she dropped into a chair. "Oh god, it was awful! I thought I was prepared, but he took me apart like a toy watch. My classmates were giggling in the jury box. I've never been so humiliated in my life."

Javeed sat up, nodding. "I remember that. You were inconsolable that night."

"And I won't go through that again," Kristine said. "I can't."

Miguel put a comforting hand on her shoulder. "Maybe you can't go through it alone. But you won't be alone. You'll be with us!"

She sighed and touched his hand. "Miguel, if you're that determined to do this, at least let me recommend someone."

"Kristine, I know you don't want to spend the rest of your life doing wills and trusts."

"How do you know that?"

"You said so last night after your second martini."

"Oh god, I get so confessional."

"I think you stay in Wills and Trusts because, first of all, you're good at it. And second, you feel safe there. But maybe it's time to step out of your comfort zone."

Kristine looked back and forth at Miguel and Javeed before she said, "You really think so?"

"Yes." Miguel held out his hands and lifted Kristine from her chair. "This is a chance to challenge yourself. Take a risk. Grow. This case will be huge," Miguel said. "You'll be setting legal precedent."

Javeed stood, saying, "And think of the publicity!"

"This could put you on partner track!"

"Oh my god," Kristine said, "I hadn't thought of that."

"Are you kidding? This is an absolute career maker!"

Kristine put a hand to her chest. "And you'd trust me with the case?"

"I wouldn't trust anyone else," Miguel said. "What do you say? Are you in?"

Miguel extended his hand, palm down, like a coach in the middle of a huddle.

Javeed stepped forward and put his hand on top of Miguel's and said, "We need you. Are you in?"

"Yes! Let's do this!" Kristine put her hand on top of the others and together they proclaimed, "*Lex clavatoris designati rescindenda est!*"

They erupted from their huddle and did a ridiculous dance that didn't seem to have been thoughtfully choreographed but was thoroughly infused with enthusiasm. And from the looks of it they'd done it before.

"OK," Kristine said, "we have two conflicting laws. The question is, are they irreconcilable?"

"And the answer is no," Miguel replied. "We just need an exception to one of the laws so I can exercise all of my rights."

"The exception being that the state allows a doctor to end your life by harvesting your organs."

"They'll never agree to that," Javeed said.

"Why not? States make exceptions all the time," Kristine said. "For example, Georgia made an exception to their homicide laws to allow physicians to participate in executions by lethal injection."

Javeed waved his hands in the air. "Why does any of this even matter? Why does the state care? He's going to die anyway."

"Here's an old law school brainteaser. A guy jumps off a ten-story building with intent to kill himself. As he passes the third floor, he's shot and killed by someone firing a gun out the window. Is the death homicide or suicide?"

"It's homicide," Miguel said. "It doesn't matter that the guy was 'going to die anyway.' The bullet killed him and that's all that matters."

"Hang on." Javeed waved his hands again. "What was the guy on the third floor shooting at?"

"Question for another time," Kristine said. "In the meanwhile, we need to think about our pleading."

"Wait a second!" Miguel pointed at Javeed. "What you said a second ago, 'think of the publicity.' Before we ask the courts for their opinion, we need to get public opinion on our side."

Javeed asked if Miguel thought there were people out there who would believe one person saving the lives of eight other people would be a bad thing.

"You'd be surprised," Miguel said. "We need to convince the public that anyone on our side is trying to save eight good people who will otherwise die. We need to explain that we're just trying to save lives."

"And we're going to do this... how?"

"Guys," Miguel said. "We're going on *Oprah*!"

***

In his defense, allow me to point out that Miguel had not watched a minute of daytime television since he was in college. So he had no way of knowing the venerable Ms. Winfrey was no longer on the air. His point was simply that if they wanted to get the public on their side before raising a legal stink about the situation—and possibly handing narrative control to whatever opposition they might encounter—they should take advantage of the reach of mass media to get their story out first.

And while Javeed and Kristine agreed wholeheartedly, it turned out that despite their collection of advanced degrees, none of them had the slightest idea where to start.

Finally, one of them ventured, "We do a press release, right?"

"That sounds right," Kristine said.

"There's probably some standard format for doing one, don't you think?"

"Makes sense," Miguel said. "Bound to be some how-to guidelines on the web."

They each jumped on their devices. Miguel had his laptop, Javeed worked his tablet, Kristine was on her phone. It didn't take long. "OK, here we go," Miguel said. "AP Style Press Release."

Kristine looked up from her phone. "AP like Associated Press? That's a bit antiquated, don't you think?"

"What do you expect? This is the guy who thought Oprah was still on television."

"Can we please move on?"

"I guess AP might still be a thing," Kristine said, "But I was thinking more twenty-first century, something along the lines of social influencers." She paused. "Miguel, do you know what—"

"Yes, I have in fact heard of those," Miguel said. "Don't know anything about them, but I've heard that term before. So, fine, you look into social influencers, we'll go old school."

They spent some time researching traditional approaches and scouring the web for tips from hot influencers. After a few minutes, Javeed said, "Says here the first thing we need is a clear message, a strong story."

"Like, 'dying man wants to save eight lives?' That seems pretty strong."

"Yeah, but that's not news," Javeed said. "Every doctor I know wants to save lives. Plus it needs to be about more than just something you want."

"OK," Miguel said. "So maybe, dying man figures out *how* to save the lives of eight others."

"That's better," Javeed said. "Maybe we should give more information about the big picture. Let the numbers do some talking. Over a hundred thousand on waiting lists, twenty-two dying every day, that sort of thing."

"There's an old saying," Kristine said. "A single death is a tragedy. A million deaths is a statistic."

"So what's eight deaths," Miguel said, "an awkward moment? Oh, wait, nine deaths if you count me."

"That's my point," Kristine said. "For the purposes of this press release, you are the tragedy. Your tragedy is the focus but we also need to shine a light on the eight deaths you can prevent if the state will simply allow you to."

Javeed looked up from his tablet. "Says here we should also make the press release visual."

"OK," Miguel said. "How about we add a picture of me standing in front of a row of eight caskets?"

"Or maybe a picture of you with eight people who need transplants?" Kristine said.

"Do people who need transplants look like they need one?"

"Good point," Javeed said. "Caskets are probably the better visual."

Kristine wagged her phone in the air. "There are a lot of these social influencers out there," she said. "But it looks like they mainly focus on increasing brand awareness about mostly useless products," Kristine said.

"Any of them focused on social issues?"

"Let's see." Kristine scrolled down a bit, reading more. "Oh, lord. Here's a story about a big-shot influencer who landed in the hospital after taking the so-called 'Toilet Virus Challenge.' There's a video of this genius licking a toilet seat in a bus station."

"Does he need an organ?" Miguel said.

"Other than a brain?"

It went on like this for a while. They abandoned the social influencer angle and settled on the old-school press release, taking a break for lunch before working through the afternoon and into the cocktail hour. Javeed and Kristine mainly didn't want Miguel spending the weekend alone, obsessing on his diagnosis. And doing this project was a great excuse to be together without indulging in a pity-party.

Sunday was more of the same. By the end of the weekend they had mocked up a solid press release. The reason it took so long to do such a simple task, as I understand it, is that they were doing a fair amount of day drinking.

By six they were wrapping up. Javeed and Kristine had to get back to work the next day, leaving Miguel to finalize the thing and send it out.

"According to this, there are two ways to do it," Javeed said. "You either label it Embargoed for a certain date or it's for Immediate Release."

Miguel looked at Javeed and said, "How long did you say I have?"

"There's no way to know."

"Immediate Release it is!"

***

At this point I would understand if you were saying to yourself, "Hey, this guy wasn't even there! How does he know what happened and who said what?"

It's a fair question. And I'll readily admit that it's true. I wasn't there for Miguel's diagnosis. And I wasn't at the bar with them afterwards, nor was I at Miguel's house the next day. But, later, when it was all over and the smoke had cleared, I talked to everyone involved and learned about what happened before I became part of the story, and I took detailed notes, which is my custom, so I am sure that I got the gist of it.

No, better than that, I'm sure I got to the heart of it. You can trust me on this. I'm a professional in the matter of storytelling, something we will get to soon enough. As I said before, you should relish the anticipation.

In the meanwhile, as I recount these moments and bits of dialogue and speculate on inner thoughts and outward reactions between the people who were part of the story, keep in mind that I may not have their words exactly as they spoke them, their thoughts precisely as they ruminated, or if they moved in certain ways and did certain things in the moment.

What's important is that—as I said at the very top—this is a story I promised to tell and I'm telling it to the best of my ability, with a few added flourishes because sometime reality just doesn't play as well as you would like.

With that in mind, let's get back to what happened next.

First thing Monday morning Miguel called into work to say he was cashing in all of his sick days and vacation time. He then created a list of journalists to receive the press release. Since this problem could be solved only by the powers that be in California and since the only citizens that could apply pressure to these powers were those residing in the Golden State, there was no point trying to engage with the *New York Times*. It made more sense to send the release to all the newspapers and television stations in California's major media markets. He also included the *Senate Daily Journal* and the *Assembly Daily Journal* in the state capital in the hopes of reaching legislators who they might engage on the subject.

Miguel then signed up with an email marketing service, attached the document with the headline: "For Immediate Release" and hit "send."

An hour after his press release went out, Miguel started to receive responses. A few replied with out-of-hand rejections. Several reporters indicated they had a mild interest in doing something on the story later in the year. But local TV personality Lynn Mitchum from Channel Six said she loved it. She wanted to do a human interest story on Miguel and his situation as soon as possible.

4

After speaking with the show's scheduler, Miguel got Kristine and Javeed on a conference call and said, "Great news! I'm doing a live interview Thursday morning with Lynn Mitchum."

There was a long pause before Kristine said, "Oh my god, she is *so* not Oprah."

"That's what I've heard," Miguel said. "But my current operating philosophy is that beggars can't be choosers. She was the only one who answered."

"In the first hour!" Kristine said. "She was the only one who answered in the first hour."

"Yeah, but see I'm running out of hours, so…"

"Sure, but Lynn Mitchum? I mean, couldn't you find someone from ISIS?"

"I know, I know, but—"

"You've got to call it off," Kristine said. "Right now. She'll eat you alive!"

"Look, we just want the exposure, right? Besides, how mean is she going to be to a guy with two terminal diseases?"

Thursday morning, Miguel drove to the television studios in Burbank, cleared Security, and was ushered into the green room to wait for his segment. A young woman came in to apply a little make up and, in the course of things, suggested Miguel might want to start using a hydrating serum with aloe water for his combination skin issue.

"Funny you should mention that," Miguel said. "I've been thinking I should take my hydration game to the next level."

A few minutes later, an associate producer stuck her head into the room and said, "Miguel, we're ready for you."

They arrived on set just as the program was going into a commercial break. The set consisted of a large oval glass-top table, about four feet high with three barstool-chairs for the host and guests. Miguel was shown to his seat.

Lynn Mitchum stood at the edge of the set conferring with her director. She was an angular blonde in her thirties, attractive in a stringent sort of way. As the commercial break was winding down she joined Miguel on the set, clipping on her lapel mic and indicating Miguel should do the same. She reached over and put a hand on Miguel's arm. "Just relax. This should be fun. I'm only half as mean as people say."

Someone behind the bright lights said, "And we're live in three… two…"

Lynn perked up, aimed herself at the camera, and said, "Welcome back, everybody. My next guest is Miguel Padilla, who has recently been diagnosed with two terminal diseases. His response to this situation is, well, to say the least it's rather unorthodox. Miguel, thanks so much for taking the time to talk with us."

He gave a nod. "I appreciate the opportunity."

"So, Miguel, if you don't mind, let's jump right in and talk about the shocking request you plan to make of the courts."

"I'm not sure I'd characterize the request as shocking when you really think about—"

"Let me clarify what I mean by shocking," she said. "Because of your diagnoses, you intend to ask the State to allow surgeons to, for lack of a better phrase, harvest you to death."

"That would be a… sensational way to put it."

"Thank you so much, Miguel."

"Not sensational like fantastic," he said. "I meant it more like unnecessarily melodramatic."

"I see. Well, how would you put it, Miguel?

"I'd say we're going to ask the state to make an exception in the law to allow me to donate my organs and save the lives of eight people who are going to die otherwise."

"My goodness." Lynn paused for a moment before saying, "Well, that sounds crazy as a soup sandwich to me but I'm no psychiatrist, so let's bring on someone who is. He's a best-selling author whose new book *Celebrating Selfishness*, is just out. Dr. Alex Pryor."

Dr. Pryor came strutting out from the wings, a copy of a book in hand. He was mid-fifties, with comically white teeth, and a suit that looked too tight even on his trim figure. He and Lynn kissed cheeks before he took his seat.

"Dr. Pryor, thanks for joining us."

Miguel looked at Lynn and said, "Are you serious? This guy?"

Dr. Pryor flashed his veneers. "Pleasure to be here, Lynn. Thanks for having me on again."

"So you've been listening to this, what are your thoughts?"

"Lynn, I talk about this condition in my new book, *Celebrating Selfishness*. The type we're dealing with is what I call a 'do-gooder.' It's a debilitating personality disorder."

"What's the disorder called?"

"Generally, it's called altruism, but in this case we're dealing with an extreme form that we refer to as pathological or cold-blooded altruism."

"Sounds horrible," Lynn said. "Can you give us an example?"

"Well, at one end of the do-gooder spectrum, you might hold the door for a stranger, even though there's nothing in it for you," Dr. Pryor said. "At the other end of the spectrum is, well, a person offering his organs to strangers for no good reason."

"No good reason?" Miguel looked askance at Dr. Pryor. "They're going to die if I'm not allowed to help!"

"Lynn, this is how it starts, by 'trying to help others.'" Dr. Pryor used his fingers as quotation marks. "Look at the modern welfare state. These programs designed to 'help others' were all brought into existence by this sort of pathological altruism. I talk about it in my new book… *Celebrating Selfishness*."

"I just finished it and I have to tell you I found it to be so profound," Lynn said. "My takeaway was that you're saying we need to think a lot less about others and a lot more about ourselves."

"That's it in a nutshell, Lynn."

"Sorry to interrupt," Miguel said, "but, what is wrong with you people? Why should we put a limit on how much we help others? What's the social good in that? I'm trying to help people. I'll be dead in six months."

Lynn turned on him. "Which begs the question, Miguel: Why now? Why not six months ago? Six years? Why not donate your organs then?"

"I was using them at the time!"

"See, all I'm hearing is me-me-me," Lynn said. "'I was using them,' or 'I want to save these people.'"

"Lynn, that's a great point. Another aspect of this sort of maladaptive behavior—and I talk about this in my new book—is that Miguel likely has a subconscious desire for fame."

"You've got to be kidding."

"See? Doesn't even realize it."

"Well… subconscious," Lynn said.

"For some do-gooders, the only way they can give meaning to their otherwise meaningless lives is by achieving fame," Dr. Pryor said. "Studies show this springs from a sense of abandonment or lingering feelings of rejection in childhood."

"So, the whole 'daddy was emotionally absent' thing. That sort of stuff?"

"Exactly. My guess is, Miguel was hoping to achieve some sort of distinction in his field. Lynn, what did he do for a living?"

Miguel raised his hand. "Excuse me, I'm right here. I teach psychology."

Dr. Pryor continued as if Miguel wasn't there. "So he probably hoped to publish important research but couldn't. And now, thwarted, he's trying to achieve fame by doing this. He wants to go down in history as a pioneer in organ donation. I suspect he's haunted by a persistent and tormenting self-doubt."

"Fame? I'll be dead! Along with eight others! I mean, for god's sake, if I ran into a burning building, saved eight people and died in the process you'd call me a hero!"

"Interesting," Lynn said. "Dr. Pryor, what's your take on that?"

"Patients with a hero complex frequently create the situation they go on to resolve."

"You're saying he probably set the fire in the first place?"

"Happens all the time."

"Fascinating," Lynn said.

"It's obvious that Miguel's moral extremism is rooted in profound self-loathing."

Miguel shook his head in exasperation. "A second ago it was rooted in childhood rejection."

"And, as we know, all forms of altruism have been shown to have masochistic underpinnings. I devote an entire chapter to this in my new book."

"Dare I point out that Dr. Pryor is a thoroughly discredited crackpot?" Miguel removed the mic from his jacket.

"Well," Lynn said. "I would point out that he's been featured on the *Dr. Oz* show."

"And I rest my case."

Lynn reached over to shake hands. "Dr. Pryor, thanks for being with us today, and good luck with the new book."

"My pleasure, Lynn. Thank you." Dr. Pryor held his book up for the camera.

"Coming up after the break," Lynn said, "skin-care guru Tiffany Ross will join us to discuss how to get the most out of your exfoliating scrub and put your best face forward. So stay tuned."

As they cut to commercial, the stage lights dimmed. Lynn removed her mic, looked pleasantly at Miguel and said, "That went well, don't you think?"

***

Miguel's drive home that day took him past Lake Balboa Park. The area was a large flood-control basin that came in handy about once a year for that purpose. The rest of the year it was a vast green space and wildlife area mixed with golf courses, soccer fields, bike paths, playgrounds, a Japanese garden, and Lake Balboa itself. It was a place Miguel had driven by a thousand times but had never actually set foot in.

But after the absurdist interview he'd endured, the irrational and illogical spectacle that had been broadcast to millions, mocking the nobility of his intentions and celebrating the idea that each of us lives alone in a meaningless world, unconnected to others and free of any responsibility to anyone but ourselves, Miguel thought a stroll in the park with other people sounded like a good idea.

He walked along a bike path for a while before sitting on a bench in the warm sunlight. Under a tree nearby, he saw a woman slathering lotion on her arms and wondered if she was taking her hydration game to the next level. Then he realized it was sunscreen and he moved to a bench in the shade.

As he sat there, watching the people and thinking about his life, he was painfully aware of the cliché of this stop-and-smell-the-roses moment. But he figured it wasn't any less authentic because of that.

Miguel wasn't an overly philosophical guy, but, like most people, he'd given life some thought. The standard stuff about why are we here? Are we supposed to do something? Or not do something? And based on what? Socrates? Jesus? A life coach session you got with Groupon?

In his six years of higher education Miguel had taken just one philosophy class. The basic intro stuff. About all he could remember at this moment was the idea that the unexamined life might not being worth living. But how much examination did you need to do? And was there an issue about the quality of the examination? If your questions were as basic as Miguel's, was your life essentially unexamined? Or was life inherently meaningless, rendering examination moot?

Besides, asking how you measured a good life assumed it could be measured in the first place, right? Doesn't it simply depend on the yardstick you choose? Couldn't you measure a hundred-meter dash in gracefulness instead of in time? If your yardstick is the accumulation of wealth and power, then kindness to others doesn't count for much. And who gets to decide which is the best yardstick?

It dawned on Miguel that he had already decided. His measuring stick was his legacy. Looking back on his life, would people say he was a good man? Would they say that if he died today? Or would they be more likely to say that if he managed to do what he was trying to?

Miguel wondered how much of life he really understood. Had he halfway figured it out? What percentage of the dots had he connected? Was there a big picture? Had he seen some of it, most of it, any of it? Would he ever know? Did it matter?

Then he heard a bell toll. Just once. For him. Clear and bright and, oh, it was an incoming text. He pulled his phone and looked. He didn't recognize the number. He read the message and thought, no, that can't be right. He had to read the message a couple of times because, well, because it just wasn't the sort of text you got every day.

***

That night Miguel met Kristine and Javeed at ICU for drinks. They took a table by the windows. The television screens around the bar showed soccer, basketball, and the sports highlights of the day. A cocktail waitress dressed as a Candy Striper brought their drinks.

"Do they still have Candy Stripers?" Kristine asked.

"No," the waitress said. "But a lot of the customers, the men, think the outfit is pretty hot."

When the waitress was gone, Kristine sipped her drink and said, "So, that had to be the worst interview in the history of television, don't you think?"

"Nothing else comes to mind," Javeed said. "That's for sure."

"She blindsided me, guys," Miguel said, rubbing his face. "Said it would be a nice human interest story."

"I told you she was going to eat you alive," Kristine said. "But did you listen?"

"OK, so Mitchum used me to help promote that quack's stupid book, but the fact is we got the word out." Miguel tapped his phone. "I've had several requests for interviews since this morning."

"OK so it wasn't a total waste of your time and reputation."

"I also got an offer for a book deal, a death threat, two marriage proposals, and—"

"You got a death threat?"

"Yeah, a couple of hours ago," Miguel said.

"Did you report it to the police?"

"Nah, what are they going to do about it?"

"Who was it?" Kristine said. "I mean, who threatens to kill a man who has been diagnosed with two terminal diseases?"

"Some guy, said he was the head of a group opposed to physician-assisted suicide."

"Too bad he wasn't from a Chinese firing squad," Javeed said. "Him we could use."

"You should report this creep to the cops."

"Seemed like a loudmouth crackpot more than anything," Miguel said. "Wound a little too tight and the subject matter just made him snap. People like that tend to be all bark, no bite."

"What about the interview requests? Did you schedule anything?"

"Yeah, doing those tomorrow," Miguel said. "*L.A. Times* in the morning and the *Sacramento Bee* in the afternoon."

"Those are good," Javeed said. "So I guess it did get the word out."

"Oh yeah," Miguel said, "I also got this." He tapped on his phone and handed it to Javeed. "A text that came in earlier."

Javeen looked at the screen and said, "Christ on a cracker!"

"Let me see." Kristine leaned over to look. "Holy crowbar! Thirty thousand bucks for one kidney?"

***

"That's a bit above market price, from what I understand," Javeed said. "But if that's the road you want to go down, I'd stress the importance of not accepting a check, for obvious reasons. It's strictly a cash business."

"I don't plan to sell a kidney," Miguel said. "And how do you know it's strictly a cash business?"

"Just what I hear from my friends in Nephrology," Javeed said.

"Anyway, what am I going to do with thirty thousand dollars in the time I have left?"

"What," Kristine said, "you think I'm working pro bono?" She was only half-joking.

"Well," Javeed said, "instead of stumbling through the corridors of justice trying to get the state to go along with your admirable, if eccentric, scheme you could take the money and fund a scholarship with your name on it."

"That's a great idea," Miguel said. "Then, instead of being known for saving eight lives by sacrificing my own, my legacy would be that I opted to commit a crime to help someone who was rich enough to skirt the waiting list that everybody else is subjected to."

"Sure, put a negative spin on it," Javeed said.

"I'm just curious," Kristine said. "Let's say he wanted to do it. Could he? I mean if it's illegal to sell organs…"

"Yeah, you bet," Javeed said. "Assuming this isn't some sort of police scam to entrap you into an illegal organ sale, all you need to do is set up what they call a directed donation. You and the recipient get together and get your story straight, something about how he reached out to you on social media with an emotional plea that moved you to an act of remarkable altruism, then you sign the hospital documents swearing no money changed hands." Javeed shrugged. "It happens."

"People don't get busted for it?"

"You'd think so, but I've never heard of it," Javeed said. "All parties sort of look the other way because, why not? Insurance companies and the state like it because a transplant and immunosuppressives are cheaper than years on dialysis. The hospital and doctors like it because it's income. Donor gets needed cash, recipient gets a vital organ. Who's going to say anything?"

"That's all very interesting," Miguel said. "But since I'm not planning to—"

"And now that you've got me thinking about it, here's something else to put on your to-do list," Javeed said. "Let's say you get the state to play along with your crazy scheme and you're allowed to donate all of your transplantable organs, you'll want to make arrangements ahead of time for your leftovers."

"My leftovers?"

"Sure, once they've taken the organs, you're still worth decent money. I mean, it's not private jet money or anything but I think you can get about four thousand bucks for a torso with legs. And a head goes for five hundred these days."

"While that seems like a good price," Miguel said, "as I said, I'm not interested in doing anything illegal."

"Oh, this is all strictly legit," Javeed said. "Body brokers are a real thing, though they hate that term. They prefer to be called non-transplant tissue banks. It's big business, barely regulated and pretty lucrative from what I've read. Reuters did an eight-part exposé on it last year. Turns out most states don't even have rules governing dismemberment of corpses. There are people out there using chainsaws on the remains of the indigent," Javeed said. "Bodies and parts are bought, sold, and leased, over and over again."

"Are you kidding? " Kristine said. "I mean, by whom? For what?"

"How do you think doctors train?"

"I was hoping they went to medical school," Kristine said.

"Well trust me, they don't let you go to work on somebody's spine after thumbing through a textbook and looking at a YouTube video."

"That's mildly comforting."

"Medical device manufacturers use parts to test their products, surgeons buy them to practice new techniques. If I had to bet, I'd guess dentists buy the most heads," Javeed said. "And it's not all medical stuff either. The military needs corpses to see what sort of damage new weapons inflict, car manufacturers need them for impact tolerance tests."

"Ewww, they don't use crash test dummies?"

"They use both. See, a crash test dummy can measure how much force a body is subjected to in an accident," Javeed said. "But unless you know how much force an actual human body can tolerate, that information is useless."

"OK, we have officially gone off the rails here and I'm calling it a night." Miguel pushed his empty glass away from himself. "Let's meet at my place Saturday and get to work on legal strategy."

Kristine fished the olive out of her glass and popped it into her mouth. "I'll bring the donuts."

***

Friday morning at ten, a reporter from the *L.A. Times* arrived for the interview. Her questions were straightforward and focused on the personal and existential aspects of the story.

Miguel recounted the details of his diagnosis and how he had come to his decision. Asked how he thought people would react to his request, Miguel thought about the range of social media comments he had seen on his accounts so far and said, "Differently."

They talked for a couple of hours, ending just after noon. The reporter said she thought the story would hit the website late that night or first thing Saturday and would be in print for the Sunday edition.

The reporter from the *Sacramento Bee* called that afternoon. The line of questioning was slanted more towards the legal aspect of Miguel's request since most of the state assembly members and senators and their staff subscribed to the paper.

Miguel said he didn't know much about the relevant law but did mention that he had aced Civil Procedure during his one year of law school. Other than that he said he knew that he had a guaranteed right to physician-assisted suicide and another guaranteed right to donate his organs. And as far as he could see, there was no good reason he couldn't be allowed to exercise both rights since not only would no one else lose anything, eight people and their families had a lot to gain.

Miguel said he had no idea if anyone had ever raised the issue before, but he thought it was a legitimate question. And, given his situation, he wanted an answer.

After the interview, Miguel responded to a few more media queries, considered what to make for dinner, ordered pizza instead, and spent a quiet night at home trying to imagine what lay ahead.

5

On Saturday morning, Kristine was standing on the sidewalk in front of her house, waiting for Javeed. She had a canvas tote bag at her feet; inside was her laptop along with a few legal pads and a clutch of her favorite pens.

Javeed arrived a little after nine. He popped the trunk, got out, and looked around expecting to find bankers boxes or something. "You need me to help carry books?"

"Books?"

"Yeah, law books, you know, for looking up... the law."

"Good lord," Kristine said. "Do you still use leeches?" She hoisted her laptop. "We've got everything we need except for donuts." She got in the car. "Let's go."

When they arrived at Miguel's house, they saw a television van parked across the street. It was the same station where Lynn Mitchum worked. Her face was, in fact, plastered on the side of the vehicle, though someone had blacked out one of her teeth, rendering her as a well-coifed hillbilly. As Javeed pulled into the driveway, a reporter and a cameraman popped out of the van, prepping to shoot video.

As they approached, the reporter said, "Excuse me, I'm Curt Kingston from Channel Six *Eyewitness Action News*. Do you have a second?"

Kristine and Javeed exchanged a look on the "Eyewitness Action News" thing. They met where Miguel's walkway hit the sidewalk.

"Are you friends of Miguel Padilla?"

"Yes we are," Javeed said.

"Do you mind if I ask you a few questions?"

"You can ask, but we can't answer much," Kristine said. "I'm his attorney and this is his doctor, so, you know… privilege applies." Javeed hefted his medical bag as proof.

"Sure, OK," the reporter said. "I'm just curious, is this some sort of publicity stunt? Or is this guy for real?"

"Did you see the Lynn Mitchum interview?"

"Sure," Curt said, gesturing at her image on the van. "We work at the same station."

"Everything Miguel said is true," Kristine said. "The diagnosis and his intention to petition the state for an exception to the laws in question. The rest of the interview was the publicity stunt."

"How long does he have?"

"Unknown," Javeed said. "Death comes on its own time."

"Can you give me a ballpark number?"

"How about sooner than he'd like?"

"Could you ask him to give a statement at some point? I tried earlier, but he wouldn't answer the door." Curt handed Kristine his business card. "Call my cell, anytime. His rules. However he wants to do it, just let me know. The public's really interested in this story."

"We'll ask." As Kristine and Javeed turned to go inside, a car pulled up behind the Channel Six van. The couple inside pointed at the house with the same excitement as someone twenty some-odd years ago coming across the white Bronco with O.J. inside. The couple climbed out of their car and presented themselves to Curt Kingston, eager for their fifteen minutes of fame.

"Hey, Curt!" The man waved at him. "Are you here about that guy with the organs?"

"That's right," Curt said. "You saw the interview?"

"You bet," the woman said. "Hey, can we get a selfie with you?" They didn't wait for his reply, just positioned themselves on either side of Curt with their backs to Miguel's house. The man made his fingers into the Devil horns sign held in front of his chest for some reason as the woman snapped the picture. "Thanks!" She posted it immediately to social media with #organguy!

"No problem," Curt said.

After the Mitchum interview had aired, the station had been flooded with calls; something about the story struck a nerve with the public, so the station had sent Curt out to get whatever he could to feed the frenzy. Since he'd been unable to coax Miguel into an on-camera interview, Curt figured he might as well get a minute or two of man-on-the-street reaction in the hopes of cobbling together a short segment for the afternoon news. "Be OK if I ask you a few questions?"

"On camera?"

"Yeah, if you don't mind."

The man and woman looked at one another like they'd won the lottery. "Sure! Where you want us to stand?"

"Right there's fine." The cameraman moved around to shoot over Curt's shoulder with Miguel's house as the background for the couple. "What brought you here today?" He held the microphone out for their reply.

The woman took the lead, saying, "Well after we saw that interview where the guy said he wanted someone to take all his organs to save other people, we, I don't know, I guess we just wanted to see where he lived."

"Maybe meet the guy too," the man added. "You know, get a selfie with him so we could prove we weren't making it up that we met him."

"What do you think about his idea?" Curt said. "Do you think the state should allow him to do this?"

"Sure, I mean, I guess," the man said. "Why not?"

The woman nodded. "I had one of my aunts die because she couldn't get a kidney, you know? Maybe if they let people do this sort of thing, I don't know, maybe she'd still be alive or something."

"She was a real nice lady too," the man said.

"I'm sure she was," Curt said. "So what would you say to someone who wanted to stop Mr. Padilla from donating his organs this way?"

The couple gave it a moment's thought. "I'd tell them to mind their own business," the woman said. "If the man's willing to go that far to help others, then I say God bless him."

"Amen," the man said. "He's going to die anyway, right? Why not save some lives on the way out?"

Curt signaled to his cameraman to cut. "Thanks, guys, that's great."

Behind them, another car of the curious was pulling to the curb.

The man asked Curt if they were going to be on tonight's news. "Could be," Curt said. "That's up to the producers in the news department. But you should tune in just in case, you know?"

***

"The circus is officially in town," Javeed said, setting the donuts and his medical bag on the counter. He jerked his thumb toward the street. "We just had a brief chat with today's ringmaster."

Miguel was peeking through the blinds at the gathering crowd. "Yeah, I can see another clown car just pulled up too," he said. "Curt what's-his-name out there tried to get me on camera earlier but I politely declined."

"He told us you wouldn't answer the door."

"Yeah, but politely."

Kristine poured herself a coffee and plucked a chocolate glazed from the box. "You guys think we need some sort of social media strategy? Or a regular media strategy for that matter?"

"What's there to strategize?" Miguel said. "To quote that mindless and irritating phrase: 'It is what it is.' It's not like we can spin it so I'm *not* asking the state to allow a surgeon to spatchcock my ass and part me out like an old Chevy."

"Spatchcock?" Javeed said.

"Split in half, down the middle, like a chicken you're gonna cook."

"I know what the word means," Javeed said. "It was the image of a surgeon cleaving you from behind that got me."

"See, that's the sort of language you might want to avoid, I mean if one were using a social media strategy," Kristine said. "I think you'd just want to put a face on it, specifically your face. It's personal and leave it at that. Besides, doing a whole strategy thing on all the social media platforms is time-consuming and we've got other things to worry about, like petitioning the courts."

Javeed pulled a glazed twist from the box, pointed it at Miguel and said, "You had any more death threats?"

"No, just the one so far," Miguel said. "Well, three if you count the ones from Lou Gehrig and the glioblastoma." He crossed to the counter and selected a chocolate sprinkle.

Kristine took Miguel's spot at the window, peeking out at the gathering crowd. "Got two more cars pulling up," she said, shaking her head. "What would compel you to go look at someone's house? I mean, it's a… house."

"People on Sunset Boulevard have been making money for decades selling those maps to the homes of the stars," Javeed said. "I never got it either. You don't have any idea if the celebrity even lives there." He paused. "Now that I say it out loud, I have a lot more respect for whoever came up with the idea."

"Here's another TV van," Kristine said. "This is crazy! I can't believe a single TV interview did all this."

"I'm pretty sure it's social media," Miguel said. "The way it can amplify a thing."

"I guess the question is whether it's going to achieve the goal we were aiming for," Kristine said.

Javeed said, "Yeah, what was the goal?"

"Get the public on our side," Miguel said.

"Meanwhile, we need to get to work." Kristine grabbed her tote bag and went to the coffee table to set up her laptop.

Javeed was perched on a stool at the counter by the donuts, checking his phone. "Whoa, dude, you're totally blowing up. You are now officially #organguy!"

"Blowing up in a good way or bad?" Kristine said.

Javeed looked up from his phone. "Some of both."

"There are people against me?" Miguel said. "Why would anyone be against me?"

"Well, for starters," Javeed said, "you're a narcissist with masochistic underpinnings and a longing for fame."

"Also, nobody likes a moral extremist simmering in a cauldron of self-loathing," Kristine added.

"Hey, let's keep in mind that I'm the good guy here!" Miguel said. "I'm just trying to save some lives."

"Oh, plus you have that Messiah complex."

"Jesus Christ, you'd think I was a suicide bomber," Miguel said.

"Alright, alright," Kristine said. "Enough. Let's get to work." She pointed at her computer. "OK, first thing we're going to do is petition the court on an expedited basis."

Miguel cocked his head and gave her a look. "That's what I said yesterday."

"And a good guess it was, Mr. Civil Procedure," Kristine said. "But now that you've inspired an actual attorney to handle the matter, you need to step aside to see how the pros do it." She gestured for Miguel to join her. "Come over here."

As he was crossing the room Miguel suddenly dropped his donut and groaned. His eyes went wide and his mouth opened as if to scream but nothing else came out.

Javeed looked up from his phone. "Miguel?"

Miguel stumbled toward the sofa, reaching out for support. His eyes were now closed tight. "God…" he moaned. His hands went to his head.

Javeed and Kristine quickly took him by the arms and helped him down onto the sofa. "Hang on, Miguel. Take a deep breath," Javeed said, as he checked Miguel's pulse. It was elevated. "Breathe," he said, checking his eyes. The pupils were normal. "It's the tumor."

"What can I do?" Kristine said.

"Grab my medical bag, I want to—"

"No, don't." Miguel waved his hands. "I'm OK." He took a deep breath and blinked a few times to clear the tears from his eyes. He tried to stand, but Javeed stopped him.

Javeed held a finger in front of Miguel's face. "Follow my finger." He moved it left, right, up, down and Miguel followed without a problem. He took a deep breath and shook his head.

"I'm OK, really. It passed," Miguel said. "It goes away as fast as it starts."

"Jesus." Kristine crossed herself and said a silent prayer. "You scared me to death."

"Take a couple of deep breaths," Javeed said, checking Miguel's pulse again. "In through the nose, out through the mouth. Nice and easy. Just take a second…"

"I'm OK," Miguel said. "Believe me, this isn't the first time. And seriously, once it's over, it's over. Just like that." He looked at Javeed. "You think there's something you can prescribe to prevent those?"

Javeed shook his head. "Not my field, but I'll check with my Neurology pals, see what they suggest."

"I'd appreciate it." Miguel turned around, looking at his donut on the floor. "Aww, man," he said. "Sprinkle-side down."

***

Miguel insisted he was fine, that the pain had passed, that he was clear-headed and ready to get to work on petitioning the court.

But Javeed was adamant. He was going to get the information he needed before he settled on his next step. "I'm calling 911 if you don't put the blood pressure cuff on right now," Javeed said.

Miguel held his arm out and said, "Fine."

BP, temperature, and reflexes registered as slightly high, normal, and normal respectively. Javeed pulled a standard diagnostic set and stethoscope from his bag and checked Miguel's ears and eyes, then listened to his heart and his lungs. He asked Kristine to take Miguel's coffee away and bring a glass of water. "Hydration is your friend," he said.

"Can I at least have a donut? Me and sugar are pals too."

In the fifteen minutes it took Javeed to examine Miguel, another TV van arrived along with several more carloads of curiosity seekers. Curt Kingston and a reporter from another station were interviewing the looky-loos like they were on an assembly line. They just went straight down the sidewalk, wading through the crowd as they milled about taking selfies and live-streaming the event.

Philosophically speaking, the crowd consisted of an interesting mix of world views from the left, right, and center. Some were drawn to the story because of the right-to-die angle. This side of the story had factions both in passionate support and in rabid opposition. Others were there because of the organ donor aspect which no one seemed to oppose. A few people had arrived with homemade signs: "Good luck Miguel!" and "I Need a Kidney" and "John 3:16."

Though no one would know this until a year from now when it came out at the trial, one of the cars that arrived on the scene that day was a brown Ford SUV. The driver was a man named Ethan Chaney. He parked two blocks away because of the traffic and came up the sidewalk, not talking to anyone, just watching. He made a point to avoid Curt Kingston and the other reporter.

It's entirely possible that I brushed past Ethan at some point that day because I was in the crowd too, waiting for my moment. But I can't say if I saw him or not. He was a rather indistinct fellow, thoroughly average-looking if I had to describe him. Given that, it's understandable that I wouldn't have noticed him but I suspect he would have noticed me since I tend to stand out in a crowd, owing to my appearance, which we'll get to soon enough.

Oh, and I should mention that it would turn out Ethan was the man who had sent Miguel the death threat.

***

Satisfied that Miguel's seizure had passed and that his vital signs were OK, Javeed packed his instruments and said, "Always safer to overreact."

"Thanks," Miguel said. "I get it."

"You sure you're up to working on this right now?" Kristine said.

"Yeah, I'm fine," Miguel said. "Let's get started."

"OK, so we're agreed that first, as you noted, we need to petition the court on an expedited basis seeking immediate declaratory relief. Thus raising the question of what is the injury in fact that you will suffer as a result of the conflicting laws."

Miguel started to answer but Kristine cut him off, holding her hand up, palm facing him, a stop sign. "The answer is you won't be allowed to exercise all of your rights," Kristine said.

"In other words, I'll be denied equal protection of the law."

"Exactly."

Javeed had returned to his phone, monitoring social media. "You're trending like crazy. If I'd known this was going to play out this way, I would have made T-shirts to sell." Javeed paused. He cocked an ear toward the window. "Hey," he said to the others. "Listen."

It was indistinct at first, but, as it grew louder, it became clear. A group of people were outside chanting, "Miguel! Miguel! Miguel!" The chant stopped after a few repetitions followed by cheering and someone honking a car horn in solidarity.

Then, someone with a bullhorn said, "God hates do-gooders!"

This was met with a loud chorus of "Boo!" Followed a second later by someone throwing an egg which hit the side of Miguel's house.

This set off a brief scuffle on the sidewalk which was met with the sudden SQUAWK! of a police siren, more cheers, and another round of chanting, "Miguel! Miguel! Miguel!"

"This is so interesting," Javeed said. "They seem a bit conflicted out there. I think I'll go gauge the mood of the crowd while you work on the legal stuff." He crossed the room, then stopped at the front door and said, "Wait! We need a secret knock."

Miguel and Kristine both turned and looked at him. "A what?"

"A secret knock for when I come back," Javeed said.

"Why in the world do we need a secret knock?"

"Are you kidding?" Javeed pointed at the door. "Because some of the people out there are psychos with masochistic underpinnings and a longing for fame and you do not want to open the door and find one of those standing there when you do, so..." Javeed improvised an unnecessarily elaborate knock. "How's that?"

Miguel held up his phone and said, "Why don't you just text me when you're coming back?"

***

"OK," Miguel said. "So, if I opt to exercise my right to AB-15 I'll be denied my—"

"On the other hand," Kristine said, "maybe we should consider a writ of mandamus."

"Is that a different way of doing the same thing?"

"No, mandamus is something else," Kristine said, logging into her computer. "I'll have to look it up if you want specifics."

"Well, yeah, specifics would be terrific," Miguel said. "You know, since the courts are kind of particular about things like... specifics."

Kristine pulled up the basics on the subject. "Mandamus is a judicial remedy in the form of an order from a court to any government... to do or forbear from doing some specific act which that body is obliged under law to do or refrain from doing, etc., etc."

She read in silence for a moment then said, "OK, none of that applies." She read some more. "Mandamus may be a... OK, blah blah blah, doesn't apply... Ah, in the American legal system it must be a judicially enforceable and legally protected right before one suffering a grievance can ask for a mandamus. A person can be said to be aggrieved only when they are denied a legal right by someone who has a legal duty to do something and abstains from doing it. So that's certainly in the ballpark," Kristine said.

Miguel nodded and said, "OK, but what happened to the equal protection petition?"

Kristine seemed tentative when she said, "I'm just not sure if that's the best route for us."

"You seemed awfully sure the last few times you said it."

"It was the first thing that came to mind," Kristine said. "And it still might be the best way to go, but—"

"But what?"

"But I'm not sure..."

"Well, which one are we going with?"

"Dammit, Miguel, I do wills and trusts! This is so far out of my wheelhouse, it's on dry land. Give me a second to get up to speed!"

He could see Kristine was stressed about it and he felt bad that he was the one causing it. "Hey, don't worry. You got this. I trust you without reservation. You are the smartest person I know. We'll figure it out."

"I don't want to screw this up!"

"And you won't."

"Are you sure?"

"Yes. And I say let's go with your first instinct," Miguel said. "Keep the writ as a back-up."

Kristine agreed that was as good a way to proceed as any. Meanwhile she was going to reach out to a law professor she knew who taught in that field.

"Anyone I'd remember?" Miguel asked.

"No, this was second year," she said as she tapped an email into her phone. "Professor Shainsky? Ivan Shainsky."

"Oh, I've heard of him. He's a hot shot," Miguel said. "I've seen him doing commentary on court cases. It's a great idea. See? You're brilliant."

She smiled at him. "You always know the exact right thing to say." Kristine leaned over and kissed Miguel on the cheek. "So let's do this." She wiggled her fingers in front of the keyboard and said, "We need to make clear that a judgment of relief would allow you to exercise both of your rights without causing injury to third parties."

"Yes we do."

Kristine held a finger in the air. "We should open with a short and plain statement showing you are entitled to this relief."

"Damn right I'm entitled!"

Kristine was about to start typing, but paused, fingers poised over the keys. "It must be pleaded with specificity and particularity." She looked at him with raised brows.

"Yes! Particularly the particularity! Now go!"

Kristine begins typing furiously. "We must demonstrate a substantial claim of unconstitutional official action! Concrete and particularized! Neither conjectural nor hypothetical!"

How she could say all that while simultaneously typing the pleading document was a mystery to me. Amazing when you think about it. In any event, Miguel was caught up in the moment and shouted, "Victory shall be ours!"

Miguel's phone chimed a text alert. He read it to Kristine, "Javeed says the crowd is seventy-thirty in our favor."

Kristine continued typing. "What's the thirty percent saying?"

Miguel tapped the question into his phone and sent it.

"Finally, and most importantly," Kristine said, "this must be so detailed a pleading that it will withstand the most vigorous motion to dismiss!" Kristine finished her work with the flourish of a concert pianist just as Miguel's phone chimed again.

Miguel read the text, "The thirty percent is saying it's God's punishment for allowing transgender bathrooms…"

"Interesting."

"And that transplants are unnatural and that I should stop making a fuss and just die."

"Well bless their ever-loving hearts." Kristine gestured at the computer screen. "OK, there's the opening salvo. Let's read this over and brainstorm before we take a stab at a second draft."

Miguel was leaning in to read the screen when he heard Javeed's secret knock. Kristine shook her head as Miguel went to open the door.

Javeed came in wearing a bewildered expression. He said, "You wouldn't believe some of the people out there."

"Do tell." Miguel tried to close the door but it wouldn't shut. He tried again but the door simply wouldn't close.

Looking up, Miguel saw the ornate silver handle of my fine walking stick blocking the door, and I said, "Terribly sorry, but if I could have just a moment of your time…"

6

Miguel opened the door and there I was, resplendent in my bespoke suit.

Miguel looked me over and said, "Who are you?"

I gave a gentleman's bow and a tip of my hat as I said, "Leonard Stratton, at your service, sir. I saw your interview and I have a proposition."

I believe they were awestruck by my appearance, though it could have been mere surprise to see someone so well dressed standing on their doorstep in Los Angeles on a Saturday afternoon. I was wearing a Hemsworth blue suit, fully hand sewn, one hundred percent horsehair canvas front, featuring hand-crafted collars with leaf-turned edges, a burgundy tie with vivid-red pinstripes, a matching pocket square, carnation boutonnière, top hat, and my custom-made silver walking cane.

As I said earlier, I tend to stand out in a crowd. Call me a fashionista if you want. Some call me a dandy and I take it as a compliment. There are worse crimes in life than being unduly devoted to style.

After mentioning that I had a proposition, Javeed looked me up and down, impressed I suspect, and said, "Do you also have masochistic underpinnings and a longing for fame?"

I smiled at this because it was an excellent question. "As a matter of fact, I do!" I said. "I'm a producer."

Miguel stood back and gestured for me to enter. It wasn't a grand sweeping gesture though it was closer to that than I suspect he would have done for someone in flip-flops and cargo pants. You see, stylishness commands respect. He closed the door behind me and I extended my hand which Miguel shook. His hand was soft and warm and he had a fine, firm grip.

Kristine approached, saying, "You're a producer?"

It being Los Angeles, Miguel added, "What, like a film producer?" No one asks if you're a television producer; it's always film.

"No. Theatrical," I replied, trying not to sound snobbish about it and hoping he didn't have a play of his own that he wanted me to read.

Javeed said, "Theatrical?"

"Yes, you know, theater. Stage. The bright lights of Broadway!" I held my hands up and wagged them slightly in the jazz-hands tradition. "That's why I'm here."

Kristine said, "Because you're a producer with masochistic underpinnings and a longing for fame?" I wasn't sure what to make of her repeating that, but I forged ahead, staying on-mission.

"Because I'm a producer who wants to tell Miguel's story. On the stage. To an audience. Hell, to the entire world!" I made some more sweeping hand gestures to help underline my point. "Good god, it's riveting!" And I meant that. It truly was. "By the way, I'm very sorry about the whole..." I pointed at Miguel, circling a finger in his general direction "...thing." I smiled sincerely before continuing. "But your story? It's the stuff of award-winning drama!"

Miguel seemed quite taken by the idea. He said, "Really? And you want to turn it into a play?" He put a hand to his chest. "About me?"

In as derisive a tone as I could muster, I said, "A play." I waved dismissively and began pacing the modest living room area as I made my pitch. "No, not a play. Something much more than that. Something grand! Something with gravitas. This subject matter is far too compelling for a mere play. This begs for a dramatic form that will do justice to this potential injustice."

"No kidding? That's fantastic," Miguel said. "What did you have in mind?"

"I'm thinking…" I spun dramatically to face them all and said, "…an opera!"

Miguel turned to look at his friends as if he'd been nominated for a Tony Award. "An opera? About me?"

"Yes and tragic," I continued, "like *Death in Venice*. Oh, we could call this *Death in Venice… Beach!*"

Javeed didn't seem to like where this was going. He said, "I'm afraid we don't have time for this right now, Mr. Stratton."

The dear doctor put a hand on my back and urged me toward the door, gently but firmly. But I wasn't that easily dissuaded. I pivoted gracefully away from him, evidence of my years of dance training.

"No!" I said. "This is too good to walk away from! Don't you see? This is the perfect story. It's David versus Goliath with some Frankenstein thrown in. Think about it! Everyone's against you. The state. The media. That so-called expert painting you like some sort of egotistical madman. Unless…" I turned and leveled my eyes at Miguel, saying, "…are you?"

"Am I… what?"

"Mad," I said. "It might be helpful."

"I don't think so."

Kristine, who I'm almost certain had been admiring the cut of my suit, said, "Listen, thanks for your interest, Mr. Stratton, but we're busy mapping legal strategy here."

This time both she and Javeed attempted to herd me to the door like some common gate-crasher, but, again, I resisted. "Wait, wait, wait! At least hear me out!"

"Hey, guys, do him the courtesy," Miguel pleaded. "I mean, the man dressed up and came all the way over here. Besides, he wants to do an opera, about… me! I say we give him a minute."

"Fine," Javeed said to Miguel. He then looked at me with measured skepticism, the way doctors sometimes do and he said, "Do you have a title for this little masterpiece of yours?"

"Yes!" With a big smile and my arms spread wide, I said, "I'm calling it... *The Organ Grinders!*"

"You've got to be kidding," was Kristine's reply, which seemed both harsh and abrupt. "Like the guy with the little monkey on a chain?"

Miguel was grinning ear to ear when he said, "I like it! It's very clever too. '*The* Organ *Grinders!*'"

"Yes," I said. "It's a musical."

"A second ago it was an opera," Javeed noted.

"Po-TAY-to. Po-TAH-to," I replied, with a little more hand waving. "Suffice to say, there's some singing." I shrugged in a way intended to make them surrender their semantic nitpicking.

"You must be out of your mind!" Kristine said. "A musical? This man's dying, for god's sake!" She looked back and forth between Miguel and me, then pointed at Miguel. "He's about to ask the state of California to allow a surgeon to kill him by removing all of his organs!"

"I know! It's fantastic, isn't it? I got here as quickly as I could."

Kristine was incredulous. "But you can't make a musical out of... I mean, like... *Oklahoma*?" She tried to belt out a line from that warhorse of the Great White Way, even did a bit of hoe-down choreography as she sang: "Where the wind comes sweeping down the plain? You must be nuts! It can't be done!"

"Listen, I know a guy who produced a musical about an exterminator," I said. They had a chorus line of six-foot-tall cockroaches doing dance numbers. It was a big hit too, got extended several weeks I believe, so this is nothing!"

Kristine was adamant. "My point is you can't take something as solemn as a man's dying wish and trivialize it by setting it to a catchy show tune."

"Trivialize?!" I couldn't believe she had said such a thing. "How dare you! Songs lift us up," I said. "They inspire! Nothing touches us more deeply than music as it transports the heart and the soul to places words alone cannot take us."

Miguel nodded and said, "That's so true!" See, Miguel understood where I was coming from, he sensed my vision of this tragedy, which is why I loved and admired him from the start.

I held pleading hands out to Kristine and said, "Does 'I Dreamed a Dream' trivialize the wretched state of Fantine's life? No! Does 'Javert's Arrival' trivialize Gavroach exposing him as a spy? No!"

"Wow," Miguel said, "so you're thinking really big, like *Les Miserables*."

"Yes!" I said, enthusiastically, before taking it down a step. "Well, like that but more like if you took *Les Miz* and crossed it with, I don't know, something… less expensive to produce, you know, a smaller cast, fewer sets, that sort of thing."

"So," Javeed said, "Like what? *Sweeney Todd*?"

"No, that was rather expensive to stage, in fact. I've been in the business for years and these are the sorts of things one learns. So I was thinking more along the lines of *Little Shop of Horrors*, but *Sweeney Todd* has potential. And certainly it's got the right tone."

"OK," Javeed said, "So, it's *Les Miz* on a budget but with Miguel's vital organs instead of French peasants?"

"Yes, but far more compelling than you make it sound." I knew Javeed was mocking me, but there was no point in letting him pick a fight until I had what I came for. And even then, why? I was sure I could bring him around in time. He was an educated man; he was just trying to protect his friend and I found that an admirable trait in a person.

Javeed took me firmly by the arm and said, "I'm afraid we're going to have to ask you to leave, Mr. Stratton." He attempted once again to steer me to the door, but I'm far quicker than I look, so I escaped to continue my pitch, careful to stay out of his reach, hands up to deflect any confrontation. "Wait, wait, wait!" I said. "You haven't even heard the opening number!"

"Oh, we'd love to hear it!" Miguel said. "I've always liked musicals."

More proof that my love for Miguel was warranted. It turned out he was a devotee of—

Interrupting my narration from across the room was the sound of an incoming email on the laptop. DING! Like a herd of gazelles hearing a large paw in the dry grass, Miguel, Javeed, and Kristine simultaneously turned to look.

The three of them rushed to Kristine's computer. I had no idea why, so I said, "I'll just wait here, then." It turned out they were hoping to hear back from a law professor by the name of Shainsky on a legal question they had posed.

Miguel and Javeed peered over Kristine's shoulder. "What's he say?"

Kristine shook her head. "It's not him," she said. "But any of you guys need a ten percent coupon for erectile dysfunction meds?"

In a moment of unwitting irony, we all stood erect, shaking our heads emphatically, "No." After which I quipped, "But there's an organ song just waiting to be written."

***

None of them seemed to appreciate the humor of the quip, so I moved on, steering everyone back to my pitch. "Please," I said, "at least allow me to do the opening number before you accost me again."

"It's the least we can do," Miguel said. "Please, go on."

Javeed said, "Miguel, you can't be serious."

Miguel shrugged. "Why not?"

Given their unbridled enthusiasm, I seized the opportunity, leaping onto the living room couch and commanding their attention. I made my hands into a frame and said, "OK, picture this. The curtain rises on a man," pointing at Miguel, "you, clinging to the edge of the Golden Gate Bridge, ready to jump. As you look down at the frigid water below, you begin to sing."

Now in all honesty I really hadn't worked out the arrangement on this song yet, but I knew I wanted it to begin slowly (adagio, for those of you who know), with the reverence due to a moment as fraught as a man about to leap to his death.

By the way, I sing in a lovely tenor, if you would like to imagine it as we go. Since this might be my only chance to seal the deal, I put my heart into it as I sang,

"When at work,
Or at play,
Hear those organ grinders say,
Have you got any organs today?"

I could see the words were reaching Miguel. But Kristine and Javeed seemed to be resisting the emotional pull of the song, I think owing to the fact that some people are uncomfortable being so close to a performing artist. All I could do was continue and hope to break down their barriers.

I reset my posture on the sofa and continued, picking up the tempo ever so slightly, injecting some hope into the melody as my character looked down from the bridge, singing,

"On the road,
On the rail,
Hear those organ grinders wail,
Have you got any organs today?"

Finally I could see a foot tapping here, a head nodding there; they were becoming one with the melody or perhaps they recognized where I'd lifted the tune from in the first place. Not to worry, I thought to myself. Accelerando! Picking up the tempo yet again, and throwing in a dash of brio...

"We need some fresh kidneys,

A lung too would be keen,
Can you spare a liver?
Or perhaps a glistening spleen?"

They were eating from the palm of my hand now, so I leaped from the sofa and began marching around the room like an amphetamine-fueled drum major, lifting my cane as my baton, fiercely energetic as I worked toward the thrilling crescendo.

"Hear them cry,
Hear them croon,
When there is a harvest moon,
Have you got any organs today?
How's your aorta?!
Have you got any organs today?
Don't leave me heartless!
Have you got any organs to*dayyyy?*"

I held my pose for emphasis, but I was spent and needed to catch my breath. I could see Miguel was thrilled, but I couldn't read the other two until Javeed said, "You've got to be kidding!"

"Well, I haven't worked out the arrangement yet, but—"

"Can you spare a… liver?" Kristine said, cruelly.

"I think it's fantastic!" Miguel said. "And very catchy." He was so enthralled he sang the line again, "Have you got any organs today?" He was positively beaming.

Kristine said to Miguel, "You think it's fantastic? I think it's copyright infringement. I mean, that's 'The Caissons Go Rolling Along.'"

Javeed said he was unfamiliar with that one.

So she sang a bit, "Over hill, over dale, as we hit the dusty trail, and those caissons go rolling along…" Kristine couldn't believe Javeed had never heard it before.

"The melody? Yes," I said, "but I'm certain it's in the public domain, so we're OK there. You see, it keeps the costs down which is very important at this stage of the game."

"So then, to recap," Javeed said, "it's not so much something with the grandeur of opera or even the gravitas of *Les Miz* so much as it's a collection of songs you've stolen and—"

"Not stolen, more like appropriated," I said.

"I think it's time for you to leave."

Javeed and Kristine seized my arms and frog-marched me to the door, all the while I protested, "Wait! You're new to the theater! This is a normal part of the development process. I have a wonderful dramaturg in mind." I didn't really, but thought I'd see if that made a difference to them. It didn't seem to.

Miguel stepped up heroically in an attempt to stop them. "Guys, what are you doing? Let him go! I want to hear more!"

Miguel and I reached out for one another desperately, like lovers being separated. "They just can't see it yet!" I said, our fingertips mere inches away. "Wait, wait, wait!"

But it was too late, Javeed opened the door and they threw me out, slamming it behind me.

***

There was no way I could let it end like this. I had come on a mission and I intended to complete it. I had to find a way back in. Fortunately there was a commotion on the sidewalk involving a churro vendor and the man with the "I need a kidney" sign, so no one was looking my way, and then I saw it, the window…

Inside, Miguel was protesting, "Why'd you do that? I liked it! I mean, glistening spleen? That's good stuff!"

"We've got more important things to do than listen to that nonsense…"

And that gave me the distraction I needed. I made my way through the shrubbery to the living room window which, fortune smiling on me as it rarely does, was open. So I threw up the sash and climbed inside, ready to defend myself as necessary.

"That was my fault," I said, brushing the dust from my suit. "I should have given you more context. I've got it all in my head but that doesn't help you, so allow me to fill in some of the blanks!"

I could see Kristine and Javeed scheming to apprehend me again, inching my way as if I wouldn't notice. So I raised my walking stick and slashed it through the air as I had my foil back in my fencing days. This kept them at bay, allowing me to continue:

"What's theater without a love story? Hmm? Depressing, that's what. So I've given you a love interest, but with a twist!" This clever bit of plotting had the effect I'd hoped for, freezing Kristine and Javeed in their tracks, thoroughly captivated as I continued: "She was beautiful and she was dying. She needed a heart and she got one! Yours!" I said, aiming my walking stick at Miguel. "And she fell in love with you. This leads naturally to a heart-breaking scene at your grave where she's singing...

"I've got you under my skin...

So deep in my heart,

You're really a part of me..."

I'm not ashamed to admit that I became so engrossed in the song that I closed my eyes, emotion overwhelming my caution. That's when Kristine and Javeed sprang, seizing me again and dragging me toward the door against my will.

"Wait, wait, wait! There's more!" I said. "Unhand me this instant!"

And again, Miguel came to my defense. "Hey, guys, let him finish! I want to hear the rest!"

Kristine and Javeed were undeterred by his plea.

"I will not be undone by you two philistines!" I said.

But my words fell on deaf ears. They opened the door and threw me out again, slamming it behind me with the finality of death.

Protesting on my behalf, Miguel said, "Jesus, guys! What's your problem? That last one was really good!"

"Of course it was good," Kristine pointed out. "It was Cole Porter!"

Standing on the front stoop, I wondered what to do next. I hadn't closed the deal yet and I wasn't leaving until I had. My guess was that one of them had the idea I would return to the window so they were rushing that way to close and lock it before I got there. So I gave them time to do that and simply walked back in the front door which they had failed to bolt, much to their chagrin. When they started towards me, I demonstrated my fencing skills once again to keep them at bay.

"Sorry about the philistine crack," I said. "I know where I went wrong, forgive me. You want to hear Miguel's song, of course. I should have started there. This scene takes place in the operating room, just before Miguel goes under the knife to make his great sacrifice. He enters the operating room in his flowing hospital gown, singing, 'All of me, why not take all of me?'"

As I crooned my variation of the standard, Javeed, clever boy that he is, was looking around the room for something he could use to thwart my defenses. Before I was finished, he grabbed a standing lamp from the corner and used it to deflect my weapon. Kristine, who I must say was far more physical than necessary, grabbed my other arm and was towing me across the living room toward the door.

I was running out of options. I had to do something drastic.

I didn't want to do it, but it seemed my only choice in the heat of the moment so, as they were about to throw me out for the third time, I proclaimed, "Wait! I'll give you a million dollars for your story!"

***

As you might imagine, my offer got their attention.

Now, in the play I hoped to produce based on this story, after my character makes this spectacular offer, I would have Miguel's character look at his friends and say something theatrical like, "Unhand that man this instant!"

What he actually said was, "Whoa! Wait a second, guys. A million bucks? Let go of him." So you can see why I would do a rewrite.

Javeed, ever the skeptic, said to Miguel, "What? Why? He's not going to give you a million dollars! You don't even know if he *has* a million dollars. And, even if he did, you won't need it because, well, you know… you'll be dead."

Kristine, being somewhat more practical, not to mention conflicted on the money issue, said, "Well now, wait a second. Miguel's going to have some serious legal bills stemming from this lawsuit, so maybe we should hear the guy out."

"I don't understand why you are so keen on this ridiculous bit of theater," Javeed said to Miguel, cutting me to the quick. "You heard that first song about the glistening spleen. If that's—"

"It wasn't about the spleen," I interrupted, trying not to sound irritated despite my irritation. "You missed the point entirely if that's what you took away from the song."

Javeed ignored my explanation. "If that's indicative of the play he has in mind, he certainly won't be doing your reputation any favors."

"Reputation? I don't have a reputation." Miguel gestured at the crowd outside his house. "Currently all I have is an unruly mob and a stupid hashtag," he said. "And even that's not going to last. It's basic crowd psychology. Sure, they're stirred up at the moment but for half a dozen different reasons, I mean there's no unifying motive to keep those people together. Trust me, they will have forgotten about this by the end of the month. Meanwhile, Kristine says we don't have a chance at this lawsuit and—"

"I never said that."

"So you think we have a chance?"

"Yes, of course," she said. "But it's true that the odds are against us."

"There you go," Miguel said. "But if Mr. Stratton tells my story, if he produces a play or a musical or whatever it turns into about what I tried to do, at least I'll leave something behind, something to show that I was here and tried to do something worthwhile."

"Exactly," I said. "If the script turns out as good as I believe it will, and if we can raise the money, and if the casting is superb, and if we find the right director and the right theater, and if we catch a few other lucky breaks along the way, you will live forever!"

They all stared at me for a moment before Miguel said, "That's a lot of 'ifs'."

"Yes, and that's not the half of them," I said. "Do you have any idea how difficult it is to take a show to Broadway? Hell, it's damn near impossible to get to off-off-Broadway. No, even *that* is understating it! You wouldn't believe how hard it is to get the artistic director of, say, The Little Theater of Modesto to respond to a simple query letter about a wonderful script from an established producer such as myself!"

It dawned on me that I may have started to come across as an embittered old has-been, which of course I'm not, so I tried to soften my tone.

"Don't misunderstand," I said. "I realize how busy these people are and how many unsolicited scripts pour over the transom every day, but I would argue there's a difference, or there should be, between a script from an established theatre professional on the one hand and some mishmash of ideas on avarice thrown together by some ex-stockbroker who decided to take a run at being a playwright one drunken weekend on the Cape." I paused to take a deep breath and remember what point I was trying to make. "So yes, the odds are against us on all fronts!"

Javeed was scratching his head. "I can't tell if you're trying to talk Miguel into or out of selling his story to you," he said.

"You're right," I said. "I get carried away sometimes. But that goose egg in Modesto should have had the professional courtesy to at least reply to my query."

"Can we get back to the million dollars?" Miguel said.

"Yes! My point is, you don't seem to realize how perfect your story is; that's why I'm making this offer! Don't you see? Your story is the first and most important 'if'! None of the other 'ifs' matter without it." I crossed the room to the television hanging on the wall. I touched the screen. "Before I saw your interview and heard what you were planning, I was in despair that I would never find another story worth pursuing."

I began to pace the room, wringing my hands for emphasis. "Day after hopeless day, searching through piles of truly wretched scripts and poring over newspapers and magazines, thinking, 'If I could just find one great story, one that was so perfect I would be willing to put myself through the constant rejection of the money people, the unrelenting torment of rewrites and prima donnas, the certain rejections from short-sighted theatre companies, all the setbacks necessary to get it made.' If I could find such a story, I would gladly subject myself to all of that and more just to make it happen."

Having said all of that it dawned on me that we had returned to where we had started when I walked in the front door and introduced myself.

"So yes, going back to your original question," I said, pointing at Javeed, "I am indeed a producer with masochistic underpinnings and a longing for fame!"

"So." I turned to Miguel and said, "Do we have a deal?"

7

"Yes," Miguel said as he extended his hand. "I accept your offer." Before I could get across the room to shake on the deal, Kristine said, "But…"

I froze in my tracks. "But… what?"

"We want co-producer credit and some back-end points." She smiled at me and wiggled her eyebrows.

If only we could avoid the lawyers, I thought. I looked to the heavens and said, "Give me strength."

"We?" Miguel looked at Kristine and said, "So, you're negotiating my deal?"

"What's the matter? You don't trust me?"

"You don't think I should hire an entertainment attorney?"

"You've hired someone from Wills and Trusts to sue the State of California to force them to let you be harvested to death but you're concerned about my understanding of simple contract law?"

"That's a fair point," Miguel said.

Kristine said she would have a deal memo for me as soon as possible, leaving some of the stickier details for later negotiation. In the meanwhile, it turned out she had received a reply from her Professor Shainsky.

"What's he say?" Miguel asked.

"That he's busy," Kristine said. "Though he did send an attachment he said might be helpful." She opened what turned out to be a page from the Federal Rules of Appellate Procedure on Writs of Mandamus and other Extraordinary Writs. "Great," she said with no small amount of sarcasm. "He did a Google search for me."

She read the document. "State the relief sought, the issues presented, yada yada, pay the docket fee… court may deny the petition without an answer, or it must order the respondent to answer within a fixed time."

"Who's the respondent," Miguel asked. "The state? Governor?"

"Secretary of State is my first guess," Kristine said. "Or maybe Attorney General."

From out of the blue, struck by a sudden and powerful inspiration, I slammed my hands onto the countertop startling everyone as I shouted, "Stop!"

"Jesus! What?" Javeed had spilled his coffee onto his trousers.

"The muse visits," I said, a wild look in my eye. "Sweet mother of Moses, inspiration has struck! I have a song! A new song for the play." I tapped my forehead with my fingers. "It's forming as I speak and we must get it down." I hurried to the coffee table where I grabbed a legal pad and pen.

The others watched, fascinated, I suspect, as they had never seen an artist in the act of creation. I had the first line down on paper in no time. I began searching for a melody to fit what I had so far. I hummed and whistled and drummed with my fingers trying to find the meter I needed.

"You mind if we keep working on this?" Kristine said, motioning at her computer.

"No. I mean yes, I mind," I said. "I need your help, a rhyme for song."

"A rhyme for the song? What word?"

"The word, song!"

"Oh, how about… bong?" Javeed said with a smirk. I could tell he wasn't taking this seriously.

Miguel quickly said, "Gong, Hong Kong, long, tong—"

"Long! Yes, that's it!" I scribbled a few more lines. I had the chorus by now. I turned to Javeed and said, "I need something medical, uh, transplant-related…"

He smirked again and said, "How about 'histocompatibility'?" He was just being difficult at this point.

"Histocompat… What is that?"

"Tissue matching," Javeed said. "But good luck finding a rhyme for it."

"Please, be serious," I said. "Uh, what about blood? Do blood types matter when doing transplants?"

"You bet your ass they do," Javeed said.

"That's perfect!" Javeed had inadvertently redeemed himself with that line. I was scribbling at a fevered pace now, words flowing like the proverbial river. "Uh, alright, I need the name of uh, the guy, the one who did the first heart transplant."

"Christiaan Barnard," Kristine said, happy she could contribute, and no doubt planning to demand a piece of the publishing.

"Yes, that's the one!" That solved the third verse problem but I wasn't sure about the overall structure. Repeating verse and chorus? Add a bridge? What about the ending? Maybe something powerful to bring home the seriousness of the issue, after the generally humorous lyrics? Yes. That was it! Problem solved, then one more line and, "Voila!" I said, tearing the page from the legal pad and holding it up for all to see.

If I might digress for a moment, I'm not sure if you know this, many of the world's greatest songs were written in this matter, in a frenzy of inspiration. My dear friend, Sir Paul, famously wrote 'Yesterday' in mere minutes. So put yourself in my shoes and try to imagine how humbling it is to find yourself joining a club of such unparalleled artistic masters. It's hard to describe and this really isn't the time nor place, so let's get back to what happened next.

I sang the song once to myself, making the necessary adjustments, then hummed the tune again as I went over it in my head one last time. Without question, it worked. I took up my walking stick, resting it on my shoulder like a baseball bat. I mimed tossing a ball in the air and swung like a home run hitter, holding my end pose for effect.

"And it's a home run!" I said. "My god, I'm on fire. Move over Lloyd-Webber, Leonard Stratten's at bat now." I pointed my walking stick at Miguel. "Get your phone to record this. We can't let it get away."

Miguel grabbed his phone, hitting Record as I set the stage. "I see this somewhere in the first act," I said, "sung by the surgeon after the diagnosis but before settling on your legal strategy. This will provide some comic relief without compromising the play's serious objective," I said. "You will no doubt recognize the melody as the venerable Stephen Foster's 'Camptown Races.' So, are we ready?"

Miguel was perched on the edge of his seat.

And I began to sing,

"Ohhh, the transplant surgeon sings his song,
Do-dah, do-dah,
A large intestine five yards long,
All the do-dah day!"

Miguel recognized the melody immediately and began to accompany me, clapping his hands like a finely tuned rhythm section. Kristine and Javeed appeared to be waiting for the next verse before committing.

"Going to stick it in,
Going to make them pay,
Bet your money on rejection drugs,
You'll live another day."

Miguel looked to his friends, trying to encourage them to join, but they were both so desperately inhibited we had to continue without them.

"Christiaan Barnard did that heart,
Do-dah, do-dah,
He's the one that made us start,
All the do-dah day."

That verse coaxed a smile from Kristine, but Javeed still refused to budge. All I could do was carry on…

"Does the tissue match?
That's the one big catch,
Blood types matter, you can bet your ass,
Get on your knees and prayyyyyyyy!"

I dropped to my knees holding the last note, eyes closed, arms spread wide. I saw Javeed smile when I delivered his line. It was a small victory, but a victory nonetheless.

Miguel was applauding before I finished. He loved it. "Bravo!" he said. "That's fantastic! That's even better than the first one. I can't believe you wrote it just like that." He snapped his fingers and sang, "Christiaan Barnard did that heart, do-dah, do-dah. That's amazing!" Miguel helped me to my feet.

"Thank you so much," I said. "It needs a little work, but it's a good start. I may want to add a bridge." I turned to Javeed, trying to win him over. "And thank you for that line about how blood types matter… you can bet your ass… that's exactly what the song needed!"

Miguel was caught up in the moment, infected by the creative contagion and fueled by the adrenaline coursing through his system. "Hey," he said, "what if the surgeon pulls a string of sausage links from his scrubs while he sings the part about the large intestine, five yards long?"

"Oh, that's good," I said. "Keep thinking." I made a note of it.

"It's not five yards long," Javeed said. "It's more like five feet."

"What's that?"

"The large intestine," he said.

"Oh, I see." I considered it, both for the sake of accuracy and in another attempt to win him over. I sang it to myself, but it just didn't work. "I'm sure you're right," I said. "But I think 'yards' scans better."

"The small intestine is five yards long," he said. "Why not use that?"

Again, I gave it some thought but there was no way around the fact that "large intestine five yards long" sang better than "small intestine five yards long" and I think Sondheim would agree with me on this one. "Factually, I'm sure you are right," I said. "But, artistic license being what it is, for now—"

"Hey! Here's a song idea." Miguel simply couldn't stop himself. He'd been bitten by the bug. He sang, "Love is just around... the cornea..."

I had to laugh at his play on words. "I like it," I said. "Very *insightful*..." Again, I made a note.

Miguel wasn't done yet either. He had one more to share. "Oh, how about a tribute to Tony Bennett?" He sang, "I left my *parts*... in San Francisco..."

I put my arm over his shoulder and pulled him close, leading him over to the counter where we could continue our brainstorming. I lived for times like this.

But like all creative moments, this one passed. And you have to let them go when the time comes, as it will. It's inevitable. Just be happy it came in the first place. In a way it's like when Miguel dies. No spoiler-alert needed here, right? The man's got two terminal diseases, after all. I mean that's why we're all here in the first place. I wouldn't be telling this story if he'd only had appendicitis. So, the best approach is to be thankful we had Miguel in the first place rather than to focus on the sadness that he's gone.

When he's gone. Later.

At the end of that Saturday afternoon, I gathered my notes and left Kristine, Javeed, and Miguel working on their legal strategy and having their cocktails. Before walking out the door I said, "Miguel, now that you're co-producing, I'll expect your help. I'll set up some pitch meetings around town and we'll see about making this thing happen."

***

Ethan Chaney's part of the story presented a problem for the play. It was mostly a matter of length, which is something I had to keep in mind both for pacing and budget considerations.

You may be interested to know that in Elizabethan England the average length of a play was about 3,000 lines, which turns out to be approximately 21,000 words. To put that into perspective for you, that's roughly a quarter of the length of a typical modern novel such as the one you are reading. *Hamlet*, Shakespeare's longest play, comes in at 4,042 lines or 29,551 words. *Coriolanus*, which, in my experience seems to run for several days, is actually a few lines shorter than *Hamlet*.

In any event, a play should be exactly as long as it needs to be to tell the story, no more. And if I included all the things that Ethan Chaney did while the rest of us were pursuing our goals, the play would have run long and slowed the pacing considerably, especially if Ethan Chaney started singing. So… instead of going into all of that, I've left him off stage and unnamed. He's in the play only to the extent that we know he's out there causing trouble right up to the end.

But length is less of an issue as I tell you the story in the present fashion. So here I would be able to tell you exactly what Ethan Chaney was up to while the rest of us were moving Miguel's story forward.

The only problem, and it's not a small one, is that I never actually spoke to the man.

Yes, I heard his testimony at the trial so I have bits and pieces of what he did and what he thought, though of course we don't know if he was telling the truth despite his swearing an oath to do so. But

80

for simplicity's sake I will proceed under the assumption that he did not perjure himself.

In an attempt to explain Ethan Chaney's behavior, the defense lawyer described how Ethan had done two tours in Iraq as part of an Explosives Ordnance Disposal Unit out of Kirkuk.

They were doing a post-blast investigation one day, after a convoy hit an IED. The idea was to get in and out as fast as possible before the enemy started lobbing mortars. But they were slow that day, or the other guys were fast. Didn't matter. The mortars hit with a shockwave faster than the speed of sound. The explosions left Ethan with some shrapnel in one leg while the shockwaves did their damage upstairs.

Negative cognitive side effects, the lawyer said. Post-concussive syndrome the experts called it. Amnesia, compromised executive function, confusion, mood disturbance, and anxiety.

Ethan Chaney took the medical discharge and went home, but he didn't work right any more.

I thought about going to San Quentin to interview the man, but it's such a long drive and, besides, investigators found quite a lot of information on Ethan's activities and analysis of his hard drive revealed even more, so, while I have a lot of facts to work with, the truth remains that I'm going to make some of this up.

All of that is another way of saying that parts of what I tell you about Ethan Chaney may not be factual, but it will all be true. As I said, I'm doing the best I can under the circumstances to tell the story I promised Miguel I would tell.

***

Ethan Chaney was looking for a parking space in the crowded Walmart lot. He'd been circling for a while before he spotted the backing lights of a red Infinity one row over. Ethan was approaching the spot from his direction when he saw a pick-up truck rounding the far corner and coming his way. Ethan put on his blinker to show he was there first and was claiming the spot. The mental health guy at the V.A. had urged him to do the things that signaled conformity when in public.

The driver of the truck, arriving second, put his signal on as well.

A unnerving rush of anxiety pulsed through Ethan's veins. He tightened his grip on the steering wheel and hoped he could maintain control this time.

The Infinity backed up in Ethan's direction, blocking him, and the truck swooped in, grabbing the space. Ethan's jaw clenched. He looked around for something he could use as a weapon. But he thought about what could happen if he got out to teach this guy the lesson he needed about showing respect. Back in the slammer is what could happen, or that madhouse, like last time. Ethan Chaney guessed his self-control was improving, but he didn't like it. Didn't feel natural.

Ethan sat there, looking around for another place to park. He was there long enough to see the other driver, a scruffy-looking thirty-something with a pathetic beard and some tattoos. *He's lucky I took my meds.* The guy made eye contact with Ethan and shrugged, like, what are you going to do about it? And that nearly pushed Ethan over the edge, but he maintained; take a deep breath and stay on the outside.

Ethan felt the rage he always did during moments like this and he let his foot off the brakes, drifting away from any potential confrontation, especially if it might involve the cops. He didn't want to end up back in court explaining the bloodshed and the broken bones and have to listen to people calling him a psychopath. Nobody likes that. Ethan would just find another place to park. It was easier that way.

He finally found a spot in the far reaches of the lot. *This is better anyway,* he told himself. He went into the Walmart and bought what he'd come for: some new socks, a sack of Cheeze-Puffs, and a four-pack of toilet paper.

He was OK back at his apartment where he didn't have any of the temptations he had on the outside. All those invitations to violence that he used to welcome. Instead, he could sit at his computer for hours on end, bold and powerful and righteous. He didn't even have to be Ethan Chaney. He could be any screen name he wanted.

He spent some of his time on the popular social media sites, explaining the truth of things to the simpletons who gathered there. But he spent most of his hours crawling around the dark web where anonymity was required.

Ethan spent his days and nights attacking people from the safety of his dark little room. Ethan Chaney was a troll.

***

The following Tuesday I collected Miguel and we went for an early breakfast at a hot spot in West Hollywood on the chance we might be seen.

Los Angeles isn't my home base, by any stretch, but I do know a few people in the business and it was possible I could run into them and turn that into something. But more important was the possibility I might be seen by someone who recognized Miguel from his now-infamous interview with Lynn Mitchum and that's the sort of thing that passes for temporary currency in this town.

As expected, I drew looks because of my unquestionable stylishness, which can be so important in this business—unless you are a star, in which case it may be more important to be seen slumming it, fashion-wise, just to show you don't care when you are, in fact, desperate for the attention. It's a funny town that way.

Over lattes and egg whites, I filled Miguel in on our first meeting. It wasn't exactly a power meeting with a young mover or a shaker. I hadn't had time to finagle one of those yet, but this would be a good place to start.

We'd be meeting with Norm Stuart, an old friend from New York, I explained, who moved here years ago, knows the territory and where a fair number of bodies are buried, that sort of thing. Highly respected in his day.

"Where do you live, if you don't mind my asking?" Miguel said out of the blue.

"I'm back and forth between the coasts," I said. "Depending on the project."

"I assumed New York since that's where theatre is mostly, right?"

"A fair assumption," I said. "But you underestimate the theatre scene in Los Angeles at your peril. Everyone thinks of it as a movie town, or did until the DVD numbers tanked and they stopped making anything that wasn't based on a comic book."

"Yeah, most of those are pretty lame," Miguel said. "But I thought the first *Iron Man* was good."

"I'll have to take your word for it," I said. "But here's the thing to keep in mind as we try to get this story to stage: an awful lot of the actors, directors, and lighting people who came here to work in television and movies started in the theatre; that's where their hearts are and that's where they work between the TV and movie jobs. So, yes, the theatre scene here is quite vibrant and that's where we'll focus our attention." I paused before continuing, "But even then, I don't like to say 'never.'"

"Never what?"

"Well," I said, "just because your story is perfect for the stage, which it is, we never want to dismiss the possibility of a television or film adaptation. Am I right? I mean, I believe in the primacy of theatre but I'm not an idiot."

8

An hour later we were parking in Beverly Hills, one of the public lots on a side street off Wilshire. "You're going to love Norm," I said to Miguel. "Old-school gentleman like myself except he's got a bit more wear on the tires. Less in the game now than he was in his heyday, but still enthusiastic and not without connections."

"So this guy's, what, an agent or a producer?"

"At this point I'm not sure what the best label would be for what Norm does," I said. "Facilitator might be a good word for it. People trust his eye for material, always have and he just wants to keep his hand in the game." Norm had essentially become a reader, one of those low-on-the-totem-pole jobs in Hollywood, but one at which he was adept. And if you are willing to read scripts? Believe me, people will send them.

Norm's office was on the fourth floor of an older building, halfway down the hallway between a podiatrist and a nerve specialist of some sort. The sign on the door said: The Norm Stuart Agency.

There was no receptionist out front, just a desk piled high with yellowing scripts and some bankers boxes. "Norman?" I called out. "You in?"

From the next room, Norm replied, "Leonard! Come in, come in."

We entered his office. I could see his head rising like a half-moon over the top of another mountain of scripts. He stood to greet us as we came in. "You old scoundrel," he said, reaching out for a handshake. "How on earth are you? It's been ages!"

"It has indeed," I said. "In fact, I can't remember exactly, but it had to be in New York, don't you think?"

"Must've been," he said. "Back when you had that tiny black box off-off-off-Broadway and I was peddling flesh out of The Morris Office, right? Last thing I remember is you working on a move to a larger venue, but then suddenly nothing. Whatever happened with that?"

That's when it came back to me. I'd had to disappear after that business with McElheny. I'll be honest with you, it was not my finest moment—but not the worst thing anyone's done in pursuit of art.

I'd been trying to move up from my forty-nine seater to a larger space with a thrust stage and, as is its wont, the issue of money reared its ugly head. I forget some of the grisly details, but the short version is that I needed fifty thousand dollars on the quick before the bank called in its note and I lost everything.

This led somehow to my having drinks with a theatre enthusiast by the last name of McElheny, who I thought might be good for the fifty. Before I knew it I'd told him all about Mr. Emmitt Carlton III, an international bond trader who was about to invest a cool million in my venture, all but guaranteeing returns on investment to anyone else who got on board before it happened. Well, one drink led to another, as it tends to, and it wasn't long before McElheny wrote a check.

The only problem was I didn't know a soul by the name of Emmitt Carlton III, let alone any international bond traders. He was nothing more than a character in a play I'd produced two years earlier. In any event, I strung McElheny along as long as I could before I finally had to explain that, tragically, Mr. Emmitt Carlton III had contracted malaria while on a safari in Africa before returning to London where he died of the ensuing complications, and all before making his million-dollar investment and there was nothing to be done about the fifty thousand. Just one of those things.

"You told me you had a contract," McElheny had cried. "Enforce it against the estate!" And while it's true I had shown McElheny a document with some signatures and a large dollar amount on it, such things are so easily created on a computer that, quite frankly, McElheny has no one to blame but himself for his lack of due diligence.

Nonetheless, I fled the city.

"What happened," I said to Norm, "was that I was victimized by a fellow by the name of McElheny, who pulled a short con on me." I hung my head in disgrace before continuing. "Fleeced me for a cool fifty thousand," I said. "The details aren't worth going into but it's my own fault, really. He made some promises, showed me some phony documents and, well, I didn't perform the due diligence I should have. The upshot is that I lost the theatre space and left town to lick my wounds." I smiled gamely, shrugged, and said, "Live and learn."

"It's a tricky business," Norm said. "Your trust is so often abused."

"Water under the bridge." Wanting to push things forward, I gestured at the scripts piled on his desk. "At any rate, I see you're keeping busy."

"Sometimes I'm surprised there are any trees left," he said. "Speaking of which…" Norm slapped a hand onto his desk. "Where is this monumental piece of material you hinted at in your email? I figured you'd stumbled across the script of the century and wanted to share the spoils with your old friend."

"No script yet," I said. "Not finished, anyway. But the rights are mine." I looked proudly at Miguel and made the introductions.

"Wait," Norm said as he shook Miguel's hand. "You're from the television interview, right? What's-her-name on Channel Six, Lynn Mitchell?"

"Mitchum."

"Yes, that's the one." Norm pointed at me with astonishment. "You've got the rights to this?" Norm's instincts were as sharp as ever. He knew the glint of gold when it caught his eye.

"Indeed I do, and paid dearly for it."

"So awful," Norm said, letting go of Miguel's hand. "Two terminal diagnoses?" He shook his head sympathetically while, subtly as he could, wiping his hands on the back of his trousers. "Sorry for your problems," he said, retreating behind his desk.

"Thank you," Miguel said, "And Leonard seems to think—"

"And excuse me for asking," Norm interrupted, "but you're not contagious, are you? Because at my age I can't be too careful." He squeezed some hand sanitizer from a pump on his desk and rubbed his hands together.

I chuckled softly and assured Norm he was safe as I prepared to do my pitch. Frankly I was using this meeting as a practice run as much as anything else. Before we stepped into a meeting with investors, say, or a star, I wanted to have at least one dry run under my belt, smooth any rough edges.

"So, picture this," I said, standing abruptly, my arms held out to the side as though crucified. "The curtain rises on a man, balanced precariously on the ledge of a building, looking down as he sings, 'When at work or at play, hear those organ grinders say...'" I did the whole number for him, then gave a breathless explanation on the fascinating legal angles, before wrapping it up with our second song, ending with the big finish on: "...Blood types matter, you can bet your ass... Get on your knees and prayyyyyy."

When it was over, Norm sat there nodding for a moment. Then a smile crept onto his face and he sang, "Can you spare a liver or perhaps a glistening spleen?" There was a twinkle in his eye when he said, "That's absolutely wonderful!"

"I was inspired," I said. "This man's story—"

"Exactly," Norm said, waving a hand at the heap of scripts in front of him. "I spend my life... we spend our lives... going through these thinking, if I could just find one perfect story..."

"Yes!"

"And you found one!"

"It's like the lottery, isn't it?" I said. "You can't win if you don't play."

Norm leaned back in his chair, lacing his fingers behind his head. "You know, I have an old friend, a terrific writer by the way, in case you're looking, had a lung transplant a year or so ago. But there was a rejection problem, then infection, then pneumonia. Then he nearly bled to death when they were treating him for that, ruining his kidneys, so now the poor man's on dialysis." Norm shook his head. "It's just awful what happens inside hospitals…"

"I'm very sorry to hear about your friend," Miguel said.

"What? Oh, no, my point is, he sued the bastards for malpractice. Settled out of court for ten million and…" Norm shrugged. "Who knows? Possible investor."

"By all means, send me his information," I said.

After a bit more shop talk, Norm stood to indicate the meeting was over. "Leonard, I think you've got a winner on your hands," he said. "Congratulations. And listen, I'll be talking to some people who will likely be very be interested in the opportunity." Norm walked us to the door. "You just better invite me to the premier, you old scoundrel!"

There were claps on the shoulders and promises to do lunch the following week and all the usual moves at this point in the dance.

As Miguel and I rode down in the elevator, he turned to me, visibly thrilled by the experience, and said, "That was great! The guy's going to find investors! This is amazing. And on the first meeting!"

I smiled and said, "Miguel, if I had to bet on it, I'd say we'll never hear so much as a peep from good ole Norm." I gave him a reassuring pat on the back and said, "That's showbiz."

***

The next time I saw Kristine, she confided in me about her frustrations regarding the legal matter she had undertaken on Miguel's behalf.

She said, "People think just because you've graduated law school, you can answer any legal question they have." By way of illustrating her point, she said you can take someone who just graduated summa cum laude from Harvard Law, ask them any number of legal questions (the example she used had to do with the particulars of Section 27 of The Merchant Marine Act of 1920) and they will not have an answer other than "I'll have to do some research."

"In other words," she told me, "someone specializing in wills and trusts is about as useful as a blind guide dog for someone needing legal guidance in issues of constitutional law."

But she was determined to help. So she took a run at one of the partners at her firm, hoping she might have some suggestions. After Kristine explained the situation and what Miguel was seeking as relief, the partner blinked a couple of times like a startled owl and said, "He wants to do... *what?*"

So Kristine was left to do her own research and she was finding no shortage of interesting avenues down which to travel. The problem (well, ONE of the problems) was that the more research she did, the less clear things became. Was this an equal protection issue or was it due process or neither or both or something else entirely? Sue for declaratory relief or file a writ of mandamus?

One thing she discovered was that she had misspoken about how the State of Georgia had made an exception to their laws to allow a physician to participate in executions. It turned out the legislature had not made an exception so much as they had deployed some verbal jiu-jitsu in writing the law itself, saying that physicians who participated in executions by inserting the hypodermic, injecting the cocktail of deadly drugs, monitoring vital signs, and doing other medical procedures, were not, in fact, "practicing medicine."

But, like me, you might ask: why would they feel the need to say such a thing in the first place? Well, the point of this particular verbal summersault was to circumvent any discipline that might otherwise be meted out by the Georgia Composite Medical Board, the government entity that licensed physicians in the Peach State and which was strictly opposed to their doctors executing murderers and their ilk. In other words, while one branch of Georgia's government was stringently opposed to physician participation in executions, another branch was so enthusiastic about the thing they codified it. Government in a nutshell.

Kristine also confessed to me that she had been playing fast and loose with the language by treating "exception" as synonymous with "exemption." Of course while both words refer to leaving something out of a group, "exemption" is *permission* to be left out that is granted by someone in authority, in the way that some states make exemptions on medical, philosophical, and religious grounds for parents not wanting to vaccinate their children against potentially fatal diseases. Another one of life's grand mysteries, but not one I have the time to address.

Now, in most circumstances, all of this legal talk would leave me cold. But this wasn't most circumstances. You have to keep in mind that I must have my eyes, ears, and mind open at all times for song ideas, clever dialogue, and plot twists. So as Kristine droned on about the entanglement of her legal issues, I began to think of a song. This one came lyrics first; I would have to find a tune to fit later. I could imagine a courtroom scene, somewhere in the second act of the play, where Kristine, sparring with the state's attorney, is provoked to song:

"He's going to die, he's going to croak,
One way or another,
All he wants is a bend in the rule,
So he can help his brother."

This prompts the judge to bang her gavel and reply:

"He's going to die, it's guaranteed,
Nothing on earth can stop it,

91

For reasons opaque the state has sued,
To demand Miguel just drop it."

Now, the jury rises as one to sing:

"He's going to die, that deal's been done,
We've sworn to do our duty,
His organs kept from your loved ones,
He'll soon be sleeping beauty."

Of course some of the songs I write won't make it into the final script, for a variety of reasons, but I'm sure you don't want me to spoil things for you by telling you ahead of time which did and which didn't, so, again, relish the anticipation.

***

At one o'clock the next afternoon, Javeed was at his desk poking forlornly at a grilled chicken salad while catching up on yet more paperwork. He would have preferred eating a double-cheese Fatburger while preparing to see a patient with genital warts over this, but in the interest of his arteries he had the salad. The paperwork was, sadly, unavoidable.

Something they didn't teach in medical school was that for every hour spent with patients, Javeed would spend two filling out forms. He thought they should add this to the Hippocratic Oath: "First, do no paperwork."

Javeed stabbed a strip of the limp chicken and held it up for inspection. He had sincere doubts about the authenticity of the grill marks striping the rubbery protein. But before he could complete his investigation, there was a knock on the door. Javeed looked up, hoping it was someone with a gushing wound or a compound fracture, any sort of medical emergency that would take him away from the paperwork. But instead, standing in the doorway was a perfectly healthy man he recognized but whom he didn't know.

The man said, "Dr. Ahmadi?"

"That's right." Javeed laid the chicken onto the bed of wilting lettuce and said, "Can I help you?"

"I'm Jake Trapper," the man said, tapping the clip-on ID dangling from his shirt. "I'm with SCOPE, procurement transplant coordinator." He gave a friendly smile. "You got a second?"

"I thought you looked familiar," Javeed said, waving the man into his office. SCOPE was Southern California Organ Procurement Enterprises, the region's organ-procurement organization. Javeed and Jake had no doubt seen one another in the hallways of Ascendant Medical and St. Luke's over the years but had never actually met. Javeed gestured for him to sit. "What can I do for you?"

Jake hesitated. "You mind if I close the door first?"

"No," he said, intrigued by the mystery. "Go ahead."

Jake closed the door then took a seat across from Javeed, glancing around the office. "Nice skeleton," he said. "The real thing?"

"Nah." Javeed shook his head. "Plastic, fiberglass, I don't really know."

"Don't blame you. Those real ones are pricey."

"That's true." Javeed nodded as he searched for small talk. "So," he said, "how's business?"

"Same as ever," Jake said. "Demand exceeds supply."

"Good news for you, I guess, in a ghoulish sort of way."

"Yeah, job security's not my biggest worry."

Javeed felt they'd played footsies long enough so he said, "And what brings you here today, Jake? I'm still using all of my organs in case you were here sniffing around for parts." He smiled.

Jake faked a laugh. "Are you signed up as a donor?"

"I am."

"Well, we'll get to you in due time," Jake said. "But the reason I'm here is I saw you on Channel Six, talking to Curt Kingston. You're Miguel Padilla's doctor, right?"

"That's right," Javeed said. Nothing confidential about that since Miguel had also mentioned him in the *L.A. Times* article. "So, did the SCOPE people send you to lecture me about the Uniform Anatomical Gift Act or something? Maybe see if I could talk some sense into my patient?"

Jake poked out his lower lip and shook his head. "They don't know I'm here," he said. "In fact, I'm all in favor of what Mr. Padilla wants to do. They'll never let him do it," Jake said with a shrug. "But I'm all for it."

"Interesting," Javeed said. "What makes you think they won't let him do it?" He leaned back in his chair, swiveling back and forth.

"First of all, the folks with OPTN and the TFOT won't like the optics," Jake said.

"Should I know who they are?"

"Sorry, it's just faster with all the acronyms," Jake said. "Organ Procurement and Transplantation Network and the Task Force on Organ Transplantation. 'Big Organ' in a manner of speaking. They've got enough problems trying to get people to sign up to donate after they've heard stories about transplant surgeons sneaking into hospital rooms to unplug anybody on a vent so they can get their grubby hands on the parts."

"Yeah, but this is different," Javeed said. "Miguel is volunteering. It's an act of altruism."

"That's another problem," Jake said. "A man dives into a lake to save a drowning toddler and dies in the process? He's a hero who did what he did in the heat of the moment. But this?" Jake shook his head. "This is cold-blooded altruism and people can't seem to wrap their heads around that. Hell, people will look at you sideways if you donate a kidney to a family member. I've seen it. There's just something… I don't know, something aggressive about it that upsets people. So a guy willing to do *this* with total calculation? Lay down on the table to be killed for the sake of eight strangers? It gives them the willies."

On an interesting side note, when Javeed told us about this conversation later, Miguel said that he thought Jake was exactly right. It was something he'd been thinking about ever since the ambush interview with Lynn Mitchum.

People don't feel bad that they didn't jump in that lake to save the drowning toddler because they weren't there to do it, Miguel explained, so they're off the hook. No guilt about what they didn't do. And they can tell themselves they would have done it if they had been there.

But the same isn't true about giving a kidney to a stranger. People could do that next week if they wanted but they don't, and they feel an implied criticism from those that do. Thus, they label the cold-blooded altruist as having pathological motivations. Otherwise, they have to admit to their own selfishness.

"So," Javeed said, "You're in favor of what Miguel wants to do?"

"A hundred percent," Jake said.

"Why is that?"

"Why wouldn't I be? If he does it, that's eight people off the lists I'm working to reduce every single day."

"OK... so?"

"So I know a guy who would like to meet with Miguel."

"A guy."

"Yeah."

"And this guy wants to meet about... what?"

"About what Miguel wants to do."

***

Much to my surprise, I heard from Norm Stuart the very next day. Seems he'd been to a charity function at the August Playhouse sponsored by some old theatre rats we had in common from the New York days. One of the attendees was Toni Bottoms, an actress whose career I launched when I cast her as the star of my biggest off-off-Broadway hit, *Sweet Fanny's Revenge*, a feminist and brilliantly avant garde (by which I mean topless) reworking of *Snow White and the Seven Dwarfs*, featuring an all-female cast.

Of course there had been naysayers—there always are—but having foreseen the universal appeal of seven diminutive and mostly naked young women (here renamed Perky, Bouncy, Jaunty, Booby, Pert, Pointy, and Chesty), who spend their days delving in the mountains wearing little more than miner's helmets, suffice to say, I had the last laugh. We had a sold-out run and more press than we could fit in two scrapbooks.

So, the way Norm tells it, he was chatting with Toni and two members of the theatre's board of directors when he mentioned our meeting and gave a quick recap of my pitch. Well, faster than you can say Lin Manuel Miranda, they were seeking introductions and less than twenty-four hours later, Miguel and I were on our way to one of the true legacy theatres in Los Angeles to meet with the Artistic Director and the Executive Producer.

I pulled a sheet of paper from my coat pocket and handed it to Miguel. "I wrote a new song," I said. "'Midnight Surgery.' The lines highlighted in yellow are your parts."

"My parts for what?"

"For the pitch," I said. I sang the opening verse and the chorus. Fortunately he recognized the tune, which is exactly why I'd chosen it. The familiarity would carry half the weight and at no cost to me. "Let's run though it a couple of times if you don't mind." I paused before I said, "You do sing, don't you?"

"Not bad, I guess." He shrugged. "You tell me."

"Fine. I'll start." We did it three times and, as it turned out, Miguel had an excellent voice and sense of pitch, and I told him so.

Miguel was exhilarated by this sudden immersion into show business. I think it served as a luminous distraction from both the legal matters and the more existential issue of his impending death. I've always said one of the keys to happiness in life is having something wonderful to look forward to. And the idea of his story being told on the stage or screen was exactly that for Miguel.

Like everyone else who had grown up in the City of Angels, Miguel had friends who toiled in the film and television industries so he knew a bit about how they worked, but next to nothing about theatre. So, as we crept down the Hollywood Freeway toward our meeting, Miguel was keen to tap into my vast pool of knowledge. He started by saying, "So, are the big theatres like the film studios who buy scripts and then produce them?"

"Generally speaking, no," I said. "Most theatres are simply dusty spaces for rent. The people who run them are grudging landlords, clawing monthly stipends from the creative classes. Producers, such as myself, do all the actual work. It's our job to find what we call the Three Ms: the material, the manpower, and, most importantly, the money," I said, rubbing my finger and thumb together.

"But," I continued, "there are a few theatres more like the film studios in the sense that they acquire the material and fund, or partially fund, the productions. And as luck would have it, the August Playhouse is one of them. So, fingers crossed!"

"I saw something there a couple of years ago," Miguel said. He mentioned the title which I won't repeat, owing to an ongoing grudge I have with the playwright who still refuses to admit that he stole the idea from me after I shared it with him, in the strictest confidence, over drinks one night at the Algonquin.

"Oh, that's a nasty piece of work," I said. "What did you think of it?"

"Depressing in an award-winning sort of way," Miguel said. "If you know what I mean."

"Indeed I do." The play, which I had conceived of as a frothy two-hander, with lots of laughs and a sentimental ending was, in the hands of this unnamed hack, a swan dive into the deep end of an Olympic-sized pool of disillusionment and disappointment. And yes, the damn thing won a Pulitzer.

In any event, for the next few miles, Miguel and I talked about some of our favorite plays and films. We had quite a few in common, as it turns out. He had excellent taste, which prompted me to ask, "Have you ever written a screenplay?"

Miguel said, "You almost have to in this town, right?"

"I'll take that as a yes," I said.

Miguel nodded.

"Let me guess," I said. "A romantic comedy-adventure piece along the lines of *Romancing the Stone*. Am I right?"

He laughed. "Not even close," he said. "It was a depressing family drama about a man disappointed that his son didn't appear headed for the sort of success his father had in mind," Miguel said. "The son sets out to make him proud by following his dreams, but the father dies before the son proves himself." Miguel paused to give me a wry look before saying, "Not that it was autobiographical or anything." He turned to look out the window before he said, "It also had serious second act problems."

So there it was, I thought. The root of the matter. The reason Miguel wanted to leave his mark. I made a note to myself about a new song for the play, father-to-son, but what was the organ link? Obviously something about the heart. Sharing one, having one? Being heartless and needing one? It was in there somewhere and I knew it. I just had to find it.

But first, the pitch.

9

The venerable August Playhouse was downtown, a few blocks from the Museum of Contemporary Art. We parked in the underground lot and were making our way to the elevators when Miguel suddenly stumbled, badly, crashing onto the trunk of a car before spilling to the ground.

"Miguel! Are you alright?" I crouched down to help, unsure what to do.

"Goddam disease," he said, shaking his head in disgust. "Thanks, I'm fine."

His expression of anger wasn't just a mask for his fear. It was quite real. I mean, how could an otherwise healthy and athletic young man such as Miguel *not* be angry about his body's betrayal? It wasn't about this stumble, of course, it was about what it foretold.

"Help me up, would you?"

I held out my hand and got him to his feet. "What can I do?" I'm helpless in situations like this. Maybe clueless is a better word. I had no idea what I should do, so I swept some dirt from his sleeve.

Miguel took a deep breath and brushed the dust off his trousers. "Nothing to be done," he said. "Thanks for the hand, though. I'll be OK."

I wished there were some way I could be of assistance. I held my walking stick out for him to take. "Miguel, would this help?"

Miguel seemed quite touched by the offer, which warmed my heart. He smiled and said, "Thanks, Leonard, but I don't think I can pull that off the way you can."

"Of course, you're right." I gave a nod. "Doesn't really match what you're wearing, does it?" I said. "I'll take you shopping for one of your own when we have a chance, something that works for you. I know all the best places."

Miguel was fine as we proceeded to the elevator and into the building. He said the loss of muscular control was like the seizures from the tumor. Periodically, without warning, down he'd go. But his attitude was remarkable, so up he got and on he went. It was the perfect metaphor for my own life and was another reason I admired him so.

Naomi Powell, the Artistic Director, and Micah Parks, the Executive Producer, were both delightful. We met in the conference room, a spacious but unremarkable chamber. Naomi and Micah were serious students of the theatre, having earned MFAs from respected institutions, but, more importantly, as far as I was concerned, I could tell they had put in the grueling hours acting, writing, directing, and hustling to get people in to see their shows. I liked them immediately.

Water was offered and accepted, small talk was made, and sympathy was expressed for Miguel's situation before Naomi said, "The timing couldn't be more perfect for this. We were talking about the need for a social issue play at our last meeting."

"The problem," Micah said, "is that the season we're looking at is already drama-heavy and all the social issue scripts we've seen so far are… deadly serious, if you'll pardon the expression."

"So when Norm told us about what you're working on, with the songs and the dark comedy, we had to hear more."

I smiled as I stood, mysteriously, before moving to the front of the room. After a dramatic pause, I launched like a rocket into the pitch. "Act one, scene one," I said. "The doctor's office where the diagnosis is revealed. Our hero is blindsided, but takes the news as well as can be expected. In the course of ten witty minutes he cycles through the five stages of grief in a manner both dramatic and comedic."

I moved several feet to my left to imply the change in setting. I framed my hands like a film director. "Scene two," I said. "A bar. Our hero having much-needed drinks with his two best friends, the doctor and Kristine, a lawyer."

There was a large flat screen on the wall behind me. I went to it, gesturing, and said, "Above the bar, eight television screens showing sporting events. But! One by one, during the scene, they switch from sports to the face of a person. Men and women of all races and ages. The people don't necessarily look at the camera, but they might. They might scratch their cheek or rub their eye or run their hand through their hair," I said, demonstrating each of the movements.

"One might have an oxygen cannula, one might have a jaundiced appearance. Some appear perfectly healthy." I positioned my hand at the bottom of the television and said, "Here, on each screen, is a digital timer... counting down. These timers will reach zero at different points throughout the play. When that happens, that person's eyes will close and they will fade from the screen, only to be replaced by a new face with a new clock."

Naomi and Micah were captivated. Naomi pointed at the television and said, "The people on the waiting lists. They're dying."

"That's wonderful," Micah said.

"Yes, and it pays off in the end too," I said. "It's not just a clever bit of eye candy for this scene. The televisions are in all the remaining scenes. The characters never comment on them."

"What a splendid device," Naomi said.

"Now before I get lost in the weeds," I continued, "I want to tell you about the songs. I've taken some well-known melodies from the public domain and rewritten the lyrics and I've done this for two reasons. First, budget." I smiled, knowing how important the money is. "And second, familiarity. The audience will already know the tunes, so they will be able to focus on the new lyrics."

"You had me at 'budget'," Naomi said, batting her eyelashes.

I could swear she was flirting, and with me; a man decades her senior. As I've said, being stylish has its advantages.

"I had a feeling I might," I replied. "At any rate, I'm sure you're familiar with the traditional folk song, 'Midnight Special?' It's been recorded by hundreds of artists I suppose, from Leadbelly to Pete Seger."

"Sure, I know the version by Creedence Clearwater," Micah said. "My dad loved those guys." He sang the one line he knew, 'So let the Midnight Special shine it's ever-loving light on me...'"

"That's the one," I said, pointing at Micah. "Well, imagine that during a conversation about organ donation; the doctor brings up the oft-repeated urban legend about the man at a hotel who meets an attractive woman in the bar who then goes back to his room and the next thing he remembers..." And here I sang:

"So you woke up in the bathtub,
Just chillin' in the ice,
And on the mirror in lipstick,
A note that really wasn't nice..."

I began to snap my fingers and encouraged them to join, which they did. Miguel joined as well, drumming on the conference room table in perfect time as I sang:

"Said you better see a doctor,
And you better do it soon,
We took one of your kidneys,
And we did it with a spoon."

This drew an animated laugh from both of them. Now, to their surprise, Miguel joined me for the chorus:

"You had the midnight surgery,
Up in the motel room,
You had the midnight surgery,
And it weren't no honeymoon."

Miguel stood to take this next verse:

"Well you got the diagnosis,
Said you need a new part,
Could be a small intestine,
Or just as likely it's your heart…"

My turn:

"Pancreatic cancer,
Gonna bring you low,
And the doctor to fix it,
Gonna cost a lot of dough…"

The two of us again with the chorus:

"I had the midnight surgery,
They shined that light on me,
I had the midnight surgery,
But I got no guarantee."

Miguel's final solo:

"Well you're yellow as a cat's eye,
And your liver's running down,
Acute hepatic failure,
Ain't no fun night on the town…"

The last chorus we slowed down a step and sang it together, and magnificently if I do say so myself.

"So get the midnight surgery,
And get it while you can,
Yeah get the midnight surgery,
Or we'll call the preacher mannnnnnn."

I'd be lying if I said Naomi and Micah weren't both visibly excited by the time we finished the song. If they were trying to play it close to the vest, they failed. They shared a look of total disbelief, a how-could-it-be-this-good expression pasted to their faces.

Naomi spoke first. "I know Norm said this is a work-in-progress, but I have to ask: when can we see the script?"

"The moment I type 'The End,'" I said. "In the meantime, Miguel's attorney is working on her legal strategy which we expect will all be handled on an expedited basis so I will be writing the courtroom scenes the moment I have a sense of the direction we're heading."

"Please, please, please let us have first look at it. I'm already casting in my head," Micah said. "I can't wait to see more."

I could have gone on, but I knew it was time to exit, stage left. Leave them wanting more, as they say. "I can't thank you enough for seeing us on such short notice," I said. "And please give my regards to Toni when you see her."

And with that, Miguel and I took our leave.

On our way back to my car I explained to Miguel that "Midnight Surgery" wouldn't actually go in the second scene since it would be completely inorganic.

"What do you mean?"

"I mean this isn't a musical," I said. "It's a play-with-music, there's a difference. In a musical, anyone can start singing at any time and for no good reason, which they frequently do. It only makes sense to have songs in our play after I arrive and start singing them, right?"

"I see your point," Miguel said. "So why did we sing it?"

"To liven things up," I said. "If you just go through the plot points one after another, people get bored, you run the risk of losing them. But start singing a good song and they're yours. And I think it did the trick, don't you?"

***

Had it been up to me, and if someone else were picking up the tab, we would have all gone to Spago or perhaps Nobu on the coast. However, since neither was the case, we gathered instead at Miguel's on Friday night to catch up on everyone's progress.

I forgot all about the celebrity chefs the moment I walked into Miguel's house. The embracing aroma of ancho chiles and cinnamon put me in mind of my time in Mexico when I worked as a consultant on the Telmex Cultural Center production of *The Producers*. The young director, a scrupulously honest fellow, needed guidance in comprehending the details of the scam perpetrated by Max and Leo. Perhaps I should have protested what this hiring said about my reputation, but at the time I was in no position to turn down any offers. Plus, I was still on the run after the McElheny affair.

In any event, Miguel had a deep pan of Oaxacan-style enchiladas bubbling in the oven, his mother's recipe which the others swore by. Javeed brought makings for guacamole, plus two large bags of tangerines, a bottle of tequila, and some Cointreau. He was at the blender making what he called tangeritas. They were sweet and delicious.

We told Javeed about Miguel's fall in the parking garage. I asked for guidance on what one should do in that circumstance or in case Miguel had one of his seizures when we were out, especially since we had more meetings planned.

"Nothing you can do to prevent either one," Javeed said. "If you happen to be close when he stumbles, you might be able to support him, but it's just as likely he'll pull you down with him, so that's your call. We should probably look into getting an ankle-foot orthosis to deal with the foot clearance problem though."

"Leonard and I have plans to shop for a walking stick," Miguel said.

"Couldn't hurt," Javeed said.

Miguel nodded at my cane. "Probably something a little less 'Puttin' On the Ritz' than Leonard's," he said. "I looked online and saw something called a Blackthorn Shillelagh that I like."

Javeed smirked and said, "Oh that's right, I forgot, you're one of the Irish Padillas."

Kristine was mashing avocados as Miguel and I regaled them with a recap of our meetings. "It was pure luck," I said. "Norm's an old theatre chap I know from New York. I had absolutely no expectations that he might be able to help in any way. But he was obviously so impressed by my pitch that he talked us up at this charity event and the next thing you know we've got a meeting with actual decision-makers at the August Playhouse, which is virtually unheard of."

"It was great," Miguel said, still brimming with enthusiasm. "Leonard wrote a new song and we sang it for them."

Kristine said, "You sang?"

"Oh, he has an excellent ear," I said. "And good breath support for someone with no training."

Kristine couldn't believe it. "I tried to get him to do a song with me once at a karaoke thing." She shook her head and pointed at Miguel. "Wild Horses couldn't get him out of his chair."

"I told you, I hate that song," Miguel said.

"What was the song?" Javeed asked.

"'Wild Horses' by the Stones," Miguel said. "Too slow for me."

Kristine served the guacamole and chips as Javeed poured tangeritas for everyone and demanded that Miguel and I sing the new song. We feigned reluctance until they begged, then we refused some more before finally surrendering to the beggars and sang it for them. And with each verse I could see them coming over to my side.

When we finished, Javeed looked utterly astonished. He said, "Took one of your kidneys… with a spoon?"

"This isn't a documentary," I said. "It just rhymes! It's funny."

"No, you're right," Javeed said. "It's very funny. I actually like that one."

At that point you could have knocked me over with a spoon. Javeed was, if not on my side, at least no longer actively opposed. That was progress.

Miguel slapped the counter top and said, "Oh, guys! You're going to love this." Then to me: "Tell them about the television screens."

As I explained about the faces on the screens and the countdown clocks, Javeed and Kristine seemed to undergo a transformation. More than anything I'd said or done since I arrived, this somehow made them visualize how the story might look as a staged event, as theatre. Until now, frankly, they had been treating me as a well-dressed lunatic with a pocketful of silly songs. But this visual bit of serious drama laid on top of the humor, this added layer of storytelling, seemed to captivate them and win them over.

"It turns out they have an opening in their schedule next season," I said. "And they're keen to see a script as soon as possible."

"Yeah?" Kristine said, "How much of a script is there at this point?"

"We're early in the second act is my best guess," I said. "So much is going to depend on what happens with Miguel's health and the courts." I turned to look at Kristine. "Speaking of which, I guess that's your cue."

***

"Well, I'd say we're early in the legal script," Kristine said, doing what I had to assume was an impression of me. "Act one, scene one: We sue for an injunction, arguing Federal constitutional due process and equal protection violations."

Miguel said, "Who's the defendant?"

"A cast of thousands," Kristine said with a sweep of her arm. "We're suing anything that moves. The California Secretary of State, the Attorney General, the Executive Management Team for SCOPE, and a dozen others."

Kristine, already a bit tipsy, finished her tangerita and held her glass out for a refill, saying, "Can a girl get some service here?"

Javeed filled her glass and said, "Proceed, Counselor!"

"Wait," she said. "First, the motto!" She hoisted her glass.

Having no idea what this meant, I could only watch as Miguel and Javeed raised their glasses and joined her in declaring, "*Lex clavatoris designati rescindenda est!*" They toasted and drank like victorious Roman soldiers.

I'm ashamed to say my Latin, once formidable, was a rusty shell of its former self. There was a time, long ago, I could translate Cicero without breaking a sweat. Now I was unable to conjure anything better than *ipso facto* and *deus ex machina*. So I was in the dark as to the meaning of their toast. I waited for an explanation but none was forthcoming.

In the meanwhile, Kristine's mind was coursing with judicial minutia and legal precedent. "I think we might get some real traction with substantive due process," she said. "Keeping in mind Lochner v. New York which allows us to show not only that there is no public benefit in preventing Miguel from donating his organs the way he wants, but, worse, eight members of the public will be deprived of life as a result of the government's actions. And that violates the Fifth Amendment's guarantee that the government shall not deprive anyone of life, liberty, or property without due process of law and—"

Excuse me. I hate to interrupt, but here I must warn you that I've taken the liberty of editing the next bit of Kristine's peroration which was a tedious treatise in deathly technical legal jargon, about the Fifth and Fourteenth Amendments to the U.S. Constitution complete with case citations and footnotes.

And keep in mind that since I was paying Kristine only the slightest bit of attention and was already working on my second cocktail, I may not recount the legal details in exactly the right fashion, in fact I may have some of them exactly wrong, but it's not from lack of trying. I hope you appreciate that. I'm doing my best to tell this story, but if a law-school-trained attorney can have a difficult time switching from Wills and Trusts to Constitutional Law, imagine the level of difficulty for a theatrical producer, even a clever one, such as myself.

It was about this time that Kristine seemed to be struck by a new idea. "I wonder if I'm approaching this case from the entirely wrong direction." She looked at her glass. "God, these are good."

Miguel said, "What do you mean, wrong direction?"

"What if we argued self-defense," Kristine said.

"Self-defense?"

"Why not? The use of force is legally justified when you have a reasonable belief you're in danger, which you are with your two terminal diseases."

Javeed said, "I think the tangeritas have gone to Kristine's head."

"Oh, Javeed darling," Kristine said. "I got you something." She raised a middle finger and offered it to him. "I like this argument," she said. "The right to self-defense is well established with advocates on both the political left and the right, so it has appeal to judges of all stripes."

"I don't see how that amounts to self-defense," Miguel said.

"That's what I meant by wrong direction," Kristine said. "That's why, instead of suing on *your* behalf, I thought, why not sue on behalf of the eight people who will die if we don't prevail in court? In other words, a class-action lawsuit!"

This, I'm quite certain, is a textbook example of why you should never let your lawyer drink while practicing law.

***

Miguel was stunned. He said, "You filed a class-action lawsuit on behalf of eight strangers?"

"I didn't really have time to get to know any of them," Kristine said. "We're sort of in a hurry to get this resolved, what with the brain tumor and all."

"But now you're not my attorney," Miguel said. "You're *their* attorney."

"Yeah, but I'm still representing your interests," she said, somewhat cavalierly. "I'm just coming in through a different door."

"And are these eight strangers footing the bill? Because I don't see why I should be forced to—"

Kristine burst out laughing. "Miguel, I'm screwing with you!"

"What?"

"Medical self-defense? Are you kidding? I may have come to this nutty bit of litigation from Wills and Trusts, but I'm not a complete idiot."

"You made the whole thing up?"

"No, actually, I didn't," she said. "It's a fringe theory by a respected law professor, if you can believe that. It's thought-provoking in an academic sort of way, but please..." Kristine looked toward the kitchen and said to no one in particular, "Have we finished those tangeritas?" She wiggled her glass.

The blender was empty so Javeed set about juicing more of the fruit.

"So, seriously," Kristine said, "Bi-Metallic Investment Company v. State Board of Equalization, a tax case from 1915, established a key point—"

Sorry to interrupt again, but if I'm going to keep any momentum going in this story, we're going to have to skip over a few of the legal details. You're free to do the research yourself, but trust me when I say Kristine's bit about U.S. Constitutional requirements in regard to Due Process is a slog you will not suffer at my hands.

Unfortunately the rest of us were unable to hit the fast forward button so we listened to what she had to say. And when she finally stopped, Miguel said, "So what are you going to do and when are you going to do it?"

"Oh, hell, I filed this afternoon," Kristine said, laughing as she moved toward the whirring blender. "California Superior Court has the papers! Now we just wait to hear from them."

You can't say I didn't warn you, right? I mean, seriously, Bi-Metallic Investment Company v. State Board of Equalization? Take my word when I say *that* won't be making it into the script. Rodgers and Hammerstein brought back from the dead couldn't bring life to Bi-Metallic Investment Company by itself, let alone paired with the State Board of Equalization. And here's something else to be grateful for: I left out several pages of Kristine's lecture on the Equal Protection angle. So, you're welcome.

The point is: legal steps have been taken. Things have been set in motion.

And now we wait.

10

Then, in answer to a prayer no one knows I said, Miguel announced that his enchiladas were ready to be served. So we moved to the dining room.

I must say that Miguel sets a beautiful table in a Pier 1 sort of way. He placed the dish of enchiladas in the center, surrounding them with small bowls filled with diced radish, avocado, salsa, and cilantro. There were separate plates on either side stacked with warm tortillas.

Kristine said a lovely grace over the feast which we then set upon like hyenas. The enchiladas were exquisite, and, for the first few minutes, no one spoke. The only sounds were those of forks clinking on plates and the familiar murmurs of oral gratification. And, of course, the slurping sounds Kristine made with her drink.

Javeed interrupted the gustatory pleasures by tapping a knife on the side of his glass and saying, "Ladies and gentlemen, I'd like to propose a toast." He held his glass in the air and we all joined him, fully expecting a heartfelt salute to his friend, Miguel. So when he said, "To me!" we were all a bit baffled.

"To you?" Kristine withdrew her glass. "Why are we toasting you? I mean, other than making the tangeritas, what have you done to earn a toast?"

"Also, it's tacky," I said.

"Look, we all got to hear about Leonard and Miguel's excellent adventures in Hollywood," Javeed said. "And we suffered through your disquisition on Due Process, but what about me? Is anyone curious about my day? Hmmmm?"

"Fine," Miguel said. "How was your day?"

"It was interesting," Javeed said. "Thank you for asking."

"Go on."

"Well, if you insist," Javeed said. "There I was, sitting at my desk, staring at a demoralizing grilled chicken salad when a mysterious man came into my office."

"Oooh," Kristine said, playing along. "And who was this mystery man?"

"A guy from the regional O.P.O." Javeed looked at us as if we understood the implications of that which, of course, we didn't.

"Organ-procurement organization," Javeed clarified. "He's a recovery coordinator, the guy at the hospital who approaches next-of-kin about donating their loved one's organs."

"Oh, I couldn't do that," Kristine said, frowning and shaking her head. "Can you imagine? Like having to ask a young couple, out of their heads with grief, if you can take all the organs from their brain-dead child?"

"Well," Javeed said. "First of all they train you not to say it that way."

"What did he want?"

"He said he wants to help you."

"How?"

Before Javeed could respond, I interrupted, saying, "Please tell me he want to invest in our play." Don't get me wrong, I have a good feeling about the play attracting investors, but where's the harm in hoping for a small miracle every now and then?

"Uh, no, sorry," Javeed said. "He's trying to arrange a meeting between Miguel and someone he says can be... helpful. He was a little vague on this point."

Miguel said, "Did he say anything about the guy who wants to meet?"

"Not really," Javeed said. "He gave me a card with a name and a phone number. Just said to call and the man would meet with you anywhere, any time to discuss your situation."

"So who's this O.P.O. guy?"

"His name's Jake Trapper," Javeed said. "I've seen him around the hospital over the years but didn't know anything about him, so I asked around after he left. He's got a solid reputation. He's very good at what he does and says he's in favor of what Miguel wants to do."

"That seems weird, doesn't it?"

"I said the same thing. But he had good answers," Javeed said. "So I talked to a cardiologist I know, deals with Jake on a regular basis. He said Trapper's not exactly a by-the-book kind of guy. He's more concerned with getting parts for the people who need them than he is about the O.P.O. rules he's supposed to follow. In fact my friend said he thinks SCOPE would have fired him long ago except that he's the best guy they've ever had. According to legend, one nurse famously said about Jake, 'That man can talk a mama out of her baby's eyes.'"

"Ewww."

"So this Jake guy was all cryptic about exactly how his friend could be... helpful," Kristine said. "Any guess what it could be about?"

"Could be the guy runs a transplant tourism outfit," Javeed said.

"Isn't that for people going overseas for the operations?"

"Well, that's where the parts are," Javeed said. "At least if you want them more or less on demand. So maybe they have a surgical facility somewhere, a Caribbean island, or Central America, who knows, where they bring donors and recipients together. For a fee."

"So," Miguel said, "you think his proposal is that they fly me to their facility and have paying customers get my organs?"

"It's either that or they've got a cure for ALS and glioblastomas which they don't, so, yeah. Presumably they'll offer to pay you good money for your parts and resell them to the highest bidder."

"Morbid curiosity," Miguel said. "What would be a good price? Organs and all the leftovers you talked about before."

"I don't know, somewhere between one and two million, maybe more."

I perked up at the mention of these large sums. "Oh! *You* could invest in the play!" The words flew out of my mouth before I could stop them.

"Are you kidding?" Miguel laughed. "You still owe *me* a million dollars!"

"Yes, well, I need an investor first, don't you see? I mean, where else would the money come from?"

"Wait, so I get a million bucks from selling my organs, then I turn around and 'invest' it in the play and then you give me back the million? Leaving you back at zero. That doesn't make even a little sense."

"You're new to theatre, so, well, never mind, forget I mentioned it. I should have waited until you brought it up," I said.

"I don't know," Miguel said. "Being an organ whore isn't exactly the legacy I had in mind. On the other hand, if the Bi-Metallic Investment Company decision fails to persuade the courts..." Miguel looked around the table to gauge our reaction. "What do you think? Should I meet with this guy?"

Javeed said, "What do you have to lose?"

***

If I could tell you this story without including Ethan Chaney, I would gladly do so. But that's not possible, so here we are. As I said before, I never spoke with this man. I have no desire to. But for you to understand what happened—and to believe it—I will have to include this loathsome person in the tale.

When the time comes, you might ask: how can you know what Ethan Chaney was thinking? I know because he bragged about it in open court. So as I tell his part of the story, I'm relying on his exact words, as taken directly from the court transcripts.

I realize some of this may read like a change in the point of view of the narration and I'm sorry about that. I would rather avoid it but I can't see another way to do this. It's a formatting difficulty given this medium. First there are his thoughts, then there are the things he typed, and then the words he spoke. And of course I'm trying to narrate the whole thing while juggling those variables.

Of course you are free to skip ahead to the next part of the story and the whole thing still might make sense. That's up to you. I understand either way.

I will put <<brackets>> around the words he posted in chat rooms and texts and social media threads. These are also taken from the court transcripts. I will put "quotation marks" around any words he said. But I'm not going to put quotation marks around his thoughts because, until he uttered the words in court, they were his thoughts and that is the part of the story I'm telling.

I warn you: His beliefs and his language are crude, primitive, and ugly. And when I am finished telling you the parts of the story that involve Ethan Chaney, I will wash my hands because they will feel as filthy as that man's soul.

Proceed at your own risk.

***

The day Ethan Chaney sent the death threat to Miguel, he had taken a break from what he called his morning troll. He had slagged plenty already, like that weepy bitch who was all bent out of shape about some abused puppies in a shelter. Screw her and all those crybabies! Ethan got a thrill when he posted that short clip of some tortured dog and they all fell to pieces. Ethan put them in their place hard and fast, and he felt good about himself doing it. Bigger, more powerful. Today he was using the screen name <<BruteForce!>>

After destroying a few more of those idiots, Ethan needed a break so he grabbed another soda and a sack of Cheeze-Puffs, turned on the TV and started surfing.

That's when he came across Miguel's interview with Lynn Mitchum, which he watched with mixed emotions by which I mean he didn't know which of the people involved he hated more. Lynn Mitchum with her fake white teeth trying to act so smart and famous. Anybody could tell she thought she was better than everyone else, so she could go get screwed sideways as far as Ethan was concerned.

And how about that Dr. Pryor asshole, the piece of crap celebrity psychologist or whatever special kind of shit he thought he was that didn't stink. Ethan just wished he could run across this pile of it in a dark alley and show him who was boss.

Ethan's shrink at the V.A. was one of those types. The kind who thought he knew everything. Thought he could tell Ethan what his problem was. Acting all superior when he tried to explain about neuro-trauma and the brain swelling after the blast exposure. He thought he sounded so smart when he said things about persistent traumatic focal cerebral vasospasm. Like Ethan didn't know all about it. Ethan was only listening to this bullshit because he had to, because of the court order.

But the icing on the cake was that crazy do-gooder spic who wanted someone to kill him and take his organs to "save other people's lives." Like that's going to make him some sort of fucking saint or something. Go back where you came from with all that! What a holier-than-thou prick that guy is. You want to save some lives, sign up for EOD work for a couple of tours, like I did. Get your ass to Iraq, find out what saving lives is all about.

After seeing the interview, Ethan went back to his cave, the dark little room where his computer hummed and he felt safe. He quickly found Miguel's social media accounts and in a matter of minutes had Miguel's phone number, so he sent him a text.

<<Nobody wants your dirty parts beaner-boy so you better shut up about all this do-gooder crap or I'm going to track you down! See if they can use your organs when I'm through with you! BruteForce!>>

The Lynn Mitchum interview had opened new doors for Ethan. He'd never thought about what easy targets people waiting for organs might be. And the whole doctor-assisted suicide thing? What was that all about? You think you're suffering? I've seen friends scattered across the desert floor, so don't get me started.

Ethan Chaney found a chat room for a support group of people who had undergone kidney transplants. Grateful kidney recipients, anxious people waiting to get one, family members offering emotional support. The perfect hunting ground.

A man in his sixties told the story of how he had been waiting years for a kidney. A good Samaritan offered one that was a match but his insurance company said it would cancel his medical if he did it, so that fell through. The man just wanted to say how grateful he was to all the doctors and caregivers who had helped him along the way.

Ethan couldn't believe this loser.

<<You make me sick you pathetic old man! You're wasting space! Nobody wants to hear your fucking sob story. Do us all a favor, just go ahead and die! You won't be missed! BruteForce!>>

After the man's sixteen-year-old granddaughter wrote a mildly profane rebuke to this post, Ethan responded with a brutal and graphic rape scenario featuring the sixteen-year-old. This was up on the site just long enough for them to read it before a moderator removed it and blocked Ethan.

But it was too late. In his mind the score was Ethan 1—Losers 0.

***

I'd been working on the script all morning and it was coming right along. I'd written the better part of a new song and felt good about the direction it was heading. But I was also feeling a bit cooped up, so decided to go out for lunch. I called Miguel and he accepted my invitation to join me.

We were at a stop light on Ventura Boulevard when a city bus pulled up next to us. On the side of the bus was an advertisement for a popular television series that was entering its final season after a long and successful run. It was an ensemble show and each ad in the campaign featured one of the cast members. As it happened, staring into our car with the most beautiful brown eyes was Rebecca Vaughn, a talented actress with whom I was only vaguely familiar.

Then, as casual as you please, Miguel said, "I read somewhere that she had a kidney transplant."

I couldn't believe it. Fortune smiling upon me again as she so rarely does. I turned and stared into her eyes (Rebecca's, not Fortune's) until they drifted away and the driver behind me leaned on his horn as the light had turned green.

"Are you sure?"

"Yeah," Miguel said. "Pretty sure."

It was so obvious, I'm embarrassed I hadn't thought of it on my own. Find an actor of sufficient fame who had undergone an organ transplant and attach them to the project, or at least tell people they were attached. It was a no-brainer.

We looked her up at lunch. Her story was far better than I could have reasonably hoped for. Rebecca Vaughn had undergone not one, but two kidney transplants. Two! I was delirious. She had been completely open about her surgeries and quite emotional when talking about what she had been through. And the more we read, the better things got.

While Rebecca Vaughn was a certified television star who had done some indie film work as well, her first and abiding love was— wait for it—the theatre. We pulled her up on YouTube. There we found the cherry on top of this sundae; not only was she a top-notch actor, she was also a singer. And a good one!

"She's perfect!" I said.

The problem was going to be contacting her. I couldn't just call her agent or manager and see if they were interested in having a meeting. Their agendas are so often in conflict with their own clients. It's not unheard of for an agency not to tell their clients about a project that would be perfect for them simply because the agency didn't represent one of the people involved. They'll deny it, of course, but I have this on good authority.

Fortunately, with social media, it's possible to get around the gatekeepers and communicate with celebrities, especially the younger ones who are so active online. In this case we found a platform where Rebecca Vaughn was particularly engaged so I posted a message to her, with apologies for doing so in a public forum.

I explained that I was a producer who had recently acquired the rights to a compelling true story involving organ transplants and, being aware of her history, I had tried to reach her through her agency, but no one had returned my call. Strictly speaking this wasn't true, of course. But I've had enough calls not returned in my day to know this would have been another one of those. And who can blame them? I wasn't the head of a studio or the current boy-wonder of a network or a streaming service, so why bother returning the call?

I asked Rebecca Vaughn for ten minutes of her time to tell her about the project. Happy to do it at her agency's office or anywhere else on God's green earth.

It was a long shot, granted, and I assumed she would ignore the message or reply with some boilerplate language; the subtext of which was to go jump in a lake, but I had to try.

So you can imagine my surprise when, three minutes later, she replied.

<<OMG! The story in the *Times*? #organguy!>>

She asked for my cell number, which I promptly provided, and within another minute I received a text from her.

<<About 100 people sent me that article! Couldn't believe it. So crazy! Where R U now?>>

I had to think quickly. What if she wanted to meet this afternoon? I didn't want to go in unprepared. I needed to do more research on Rebecca's theatre work and I wanted, at the very least, to finish the new song before we met. So I replied:

<<LAX, on the tarmac, seat 3B to be specific, on way to NY. Back in 2 days.>> First of all I wanted her to see me as going First Class. One wants to make a good first impression, after all. And the two days would buy plenty of time.

<<Will arrange meeting at CIA for Thursday. Good for u?>> CIA was Creative International Agency, one of the big three talent stables in Los Angeles.

<<Perfect. Thanks so much. Looking forward to meeting you. Ciao!>>

***

Creative International Agency occupied several floors of an office tower in Century City. Miguel and I were met by a young man in the lobby and escorted us upstairs for our meeting.

Rebecca Vaughn and her agent were waiting in a conference room. Before anyone could start making introductions, Rebecca sprang from her chair and went to Miguel. He put a hand out to greet her but she enveloped him in a warm hug.

"Miguel, I am so honored to meet you," she said, breaking the embrace and taking both his hands. "I'm so sorry for what you're going through and I think what you're trying to do is, I don't know, it's saintly." She was looking into his eyes as she continued, "I wouldn't be here if someone hadn't given me a part of themselves." She wiped a tear from her eye. "Oh, god, sorry, it's emotional for me."

Miguel took it all in his stride, saying, "It's OK." And then he hugged her. "I'm glad you're healthy and I hope I get the chance to do that for someone else."

Rebecca stepped back and said, "And you must be Leonard Stratten. So nice to meet you." We shook hands as she looked me up and down. "I do love a snappy dresser. That is very smart."

I smiled and gave the slightest nod. "Fashions fade, but style is eternal." I gestured at her shoes. "And I see we're on the same page."

"Yes." She struck a pose and said, "I firmly believe that with the right footwear one can rule the world."

"Ah, the Divine Miss M," I said, recognizing the quote. "We chummed around a bit back in the Continental Bathhouse days."

"She's one of my role models," Rebecca said. "She sings, she acts, she tells dirty jokes…" Rebecca turned to introduce her agent. "Leonard, Miguel, this is Robin Harris."

We made small talk for a bit before Rebecca looked to Miguel and said, "It must be strange to be doing this, I mean, working on a project about how you… well, how you died."

"It's a bit of an out-of-body experience," Miguel said. "But it's weirdly fun too, just like Leonard." He looked at me with a smile. "He's come up with a great mix of comedy and songs and—"

"Comedy and songs? There are songs? I thought this was going to be…" Rebecca paused, looked at her agent, then back at Miguel. "Well, actually I guess I had no idea what I thought it was going to be. Pitch away!"

I stood and held my hands up, palms out, as if showing her a stage. "It's a tragicomedy in two acts with some singing," I said. "Act one, scene one, a man standing at the edge of a cliff…"

As I pitched the story, Rebecca's agent cycled through a series of enthusiastic expressions, but I could see her calculating the lost commissions if Rebecca chose to do a play over the same period of time she could be shooting a film.

After describing the first three scenes, Rebecca held up a hand to stop me.

"The television screens are such a great idea," she said. "The seriousness of them dying as they watch the dark comedy playing out below them. I'm loving this." She looked to her agent who gamely feigned an expression of agreement. Rebecca looked back to me and said, "Could we hear one of the songs… please?"

"Of course," I said. "I finished a new one yesterday and we practiced it on the way over, just for you." Miguel and I moved to the front of the room. "So, are you familiar with the traditional folk song 'Low Bridge' or, as it's sometimes called, 'The Erie Canal' song?" I sang the familiar chorus, "Low bridge, everybody down, low bridge we're coming to a town…"

"Yes! Springsteen did that on the Seeger Sessions."

"Excellent, so in this scene," I said, "we'll see someone who ended up on the waiting list. The setting is a shabby tattoo parlor, a young woman, her sleeve rolled up for the strung-out tattoo artist, begins to have second thoughts as a leathery husk of a man sitting off to the side, begins to sing…

"I got an old liver and it's turning brown,
Fifteen months of waiting around.
It won't be long 'till the burying ground,
Fifteen months of waiting around."

Rebecca's jaw dropped, just as Leonard had hoped. His research had paid off.

"The needle wasn't sterilized,
And hygiene went unemphasized.
Hepatitis C g'tting' outta hand,
Leavin' me with a withered gland."

Miguel and I belted out the chorus.

"No parts, anywhere in town!
No parts, and the number's going down!
And you'll always need a kidney,
More than you'll need a crown,
Fifteen months of waiting around."

I took this next bit as a solo.

"They got a long list for livers,

And a longer one for lungs,
No point in gettin' on it,
Unless you're young."
Again, the two of us.
"No parts, anywhere in town!
No parts, and the number's going down!
And you'll always need a kidney,
More than you'll need a crown,
Fifteen months... of waiting around..."
Rebecca and her agent gave enthusiastic applause as we took exaggerated bows. "Oh my god, that is so freaky!" Rebecca said. "I was on the waiting list for exactly fifteen months! Did you know that?"

"It's as if I wrote the song for you," I said. "Which of course I did." Her fifteen months on the list was something I had picked up during my research.

"The waiting was the hardest part, I think," Rebecca said. "The uncertainty, day after day. Every time your phone rings, you think... Maybe this is it! And then it isn't... until one day it is." Rebecca looked at the ceiling as she had an idea. "Hey, what if the people on the TV screens joined in on the chorus, you know, since they're the ones who are waiting, right?"

"Yes! That's excellent," I said, wishing I had thought of it. "And it's a nice surprise after they've been silent for so long. I like that."

Rebecca smiled broadly. "This could be the perfect palate cleanser for me. Before you got here, we were talking about how the series has been great but after all these years it's gotten too safe, too easy, you know? You flub a line? Who cares? Do a retake. I don't want to lose my chops," she said. "Being on stage is like going to the gym for an actor, it keeps you sharp."

"So true," I said. "And while we're very excited to have the August Playhouse on board—"

"Really?" Robin sounded surprised. "That's impressive."

"Yes, Naomi and Micah are very excited about it," I said. "But we don't want to limit ourselves, do we? I mean, if we play our cards right this could go the same route as, say, *My Big Fat Greek Wedding*."

"Which started as a play," Robin said. "Then spun off to be a feature." She began to see the possibilities. "To which there was a sequel and a television series spin-off," she said. "Interesting."

"How does it end?" Rebecca asked.

"We don't know yet," I replied.

"Well, we know," Miguel said. "We just don't have all the details."

11

Miguel used the end-to-end encryption app to send a message to the number on the card. Miguel said he wanted to meet, suggesting Lake Balboa Park, the building where they rent the golf clubs. He said: <<I'll be wearing a Grateful Dead T-shirt.>>

<<See you there.>>

Miguel arrived a few minutes early. As he approached, a man in his mid-fifties wearing tan slacks, a light-blue Polo shirt and a white sun visor waved him over. "Mr. Padilla?"

"Just Miguel is fine."

"Miguel, OK," the man said. "Thanks for getting in touch. I'm sorry about your circumstances. I'm Mr. Kaye."

"Thanks," Miguel said. "So like the letter K or—"

"Like the actor, Danny Kaye," he said. "You're probably too young to remember him. It's K-A-Y-E." He motioned at the two push carts loaded with full sets of clubs that were parked a few feet away. "You play?"

"Not really," Miguel said.

"Perfect. We'll just walk the course if that's alright."

"It's a nice day, why not?"

They took the push carts and headed down the path toward the first tee. "So, I saw the story in the *Times*," Mr. Kaye said. "I have to say I was both intrigued and impressed by your decision. Very noble of you."

"Yeah, well, I'm an avid recycler," Miguel said. "I'd hate to see my useful parts go to waste."

They arrived at the first tee and Mr. Kaye pulled a three wood from the bag. "Just want to make it look good." He pretended to tee a ball and, after a couple of practices, took a nice full swing. Then he slipped the club back into the bag and grabbed his push cart. "Shall we?"

As they walked together down the middle of the fairway, Miguel said, "So what exactly do you do?"

"Well, usually I connect wealthy people who need a kidney with less-wealthy people who are willing to sell one."

"So you arrange those, uh, what are they called, bogus directed donations?" He remembered Javeed talking about those.

"No, you only need to do that if you're doing the transplant in a… regular hospital," Mr. Kaye said. "Our facility isn't one of those."

"Yeah, Javeed was guessing it was—"

"Wait." Mr. Kaye stopped. "Who is Javeed?"

"My doctor," Miguel said. "The guy Jake Trapper talked to."

"Oh, OK." Mr. Kaye continued walking down the fairway.

"Javeed's guess was that you operate a transplant tourism company," Miguel said. "And you maybe had a facility in the Caribbean or Central America."

"Well, it's a tourism outfit only for those who travel here for one of our transplants," Mr. Kaye said. "Our facility is here in Southern California."

They arrived at the green. Mr. Kaye pulled the putter from his bag and dropped a ball about fifteen feet from the hole. "You a betting man?"

Miguel shook his head. "This feels too much like a set-up."

Mr. Kaye lined up the shot and dropped it in the cup. "Ha," he said. "Pure luck." They turned and headed for the second tee.

Miguel said, "So how do you usually find your donors? I'm guessing most of them don't have their stories in the paper."

"Let's just say it's not at all difficult to find people who are in need of money," Mr. Kaye said. He pointed to a bench in the shade between the second tee and the eighteenth green. "You mind if we continue this over there? Let these others play through."

They moved to the shade and parked their clubs, sitting on either end of the bench.

"So," Miguel said, "Obviously I want to donate a lot more than just a kidney."

"Yes, that's what caught our attention."

"And it's something you would be able to do?"

"Yes," Mr. Kaye said. "I wouldn't have reached out otherwise. And while I can't go into any detail, suffice it to say you wouldn't actually be the first person to donate... so generously."

"Really? Like—"

"Trust me on this," Mr. Kaye said. "Just don't ask me any questions."

"OK, so cutting to the chase," Miguel said. "You wanted to meet to see if I would be interested in making a deal to sell you all my... assets?"

"That's correct," Mr. Kaye said.

"You understand this is just my fallback position, right?" Miguel said. "In case the courts reject my case."

"Of course. I understand and respect that," Mr. Kaye said. "I just wanted to let you know you could still help others, even if the court case doesn't work out."

"Right, that's good to know."

"Can I ask, did you have a dollar figure in mind?"

Miguel hesitated. He remembered Javeed's guess that the number might be anywhere from one to two million. But Miguel was the kind of guy who had never sold an old car without looking up its Blue Book value and checking prices on multiple websites before making a deal. So he wanted to do some more research before answering. After a moment he said, "I tell you what, let's not talk price right now. I need to think about this some more."

"I understand," Mr. Kaye said. "And if you'd like to see our facility, just text me and I'll arrange it."

"Great. I'll do that."

Mr. Kaye stood and grabbed his push cart. "Shall we head back?" Miguel joined him on the cart path. After a bit, Mr. Kaye said, "So, Miguel, I'm curious. If it's not too personal, what are you doing with your remaining time? You're obviously not spending it with your family."

Miguel looked at him warily. "Why do you say that?"

"You don't have any family," Mr. Kaye said, matter-of-factly. "Sorry, I don't mean to sound callous. It's just that we don't meet with anyone until we've done a thorough background check. We're very security conscious."

"I guess that makes sense," Miguel said. "Believe it or not, I'm working with a producer to get a play or a film made about my story."

"How very L.A. And how's that going?"

"Surprisingly well," Miguel said. "We've got interest from the August Playhouse and the actress Rebecca Vaughn wants to be in it. So now we're looking for investors."

Mr. Kaye seemed genuinely intrigued by this. "You don't say."

"Oh, but I do."

"Odd as this may sound," Mr. Kaye said, "I just might know someone."

"Really? Who?"

"Well, let's say he's a very wealthy businessman."

"A wealthy businessman you sold a kidney to?"

"No, but he could afford that plus a lot more," Mr. Kaye said. "If you'd like, I can ask if he might be interested in your project."

"Sure, why not?"

They left the push carts at the return window. Mr. Kaye shook hands with Miguel and said, "So, let's stay in touch on both counts."

***

I was eager to hear about the meeting with the mystery man. I had begged Miguel to let me join him, not wanting to miss an opportunity for possible new material, but the man had insisted Miguel come alone.

So I spent the day working on the script, looking for a way to use whatever might come of the meeting. The problem was, I couldn't find one. I don't know if I was too attached to my preconceived notion of the script or if my instincts were, as usual, spot on. Normally I would welcome a twist as surprising and salacious as this one appeared to be and perhaps I could still find a way to use it, but the fact of the matter was, assuming a certain number of pages for the courtroom scenes, adding this subplot would simply make the script too long.

Still, I remained hopeful that something good would come from it.

Kristine invited us to dinner at her place for what was becoming our customary weekend gathering. She ordered some Indian food and we were having drinks while we waited for the delivery.

"He didn't offer a first name," Miguel said. "Last name only, Mr. Kaye, K-A-Y-E. Perfectly nice guy, no pressure, nothing weird at all except for the fact we were talking about a deal to sell all of my organs." Miguel shook his head in wonder that he had even uttered the sentence. "He invited me to take a look at their facility which is somewhere in Southern California." Miguel pointed at Javeed and said, "I asked if I could bring you along since I wouldn't know if the place had the right equipment for the job and he was OK with that. You interested?"

"That could be very educational," Javeed said. "It could also just be a trap to harvest both of us." He paused and sipped his drink. "Oh, what the hell, I'm in."

"Great, I'll schedule it."

Kristine asked if Miguel had negotiated a price.

"No," Miguel said. "I told him I wanted to see how things played out with the state before we talked money. I take it there's no word from the court?"

"Crickets so far," Kristine said. "I suspect we'll hear this coming week."

I suppose I shouldn't have been surprised at what happened next, but the discussion about the mysterious facility and the services they provided and the negotiations about the value of Miguel's parts started to tickle my creative antennae. The more they talked, the more possibilities began to reveal themselves. I was beginning to see there might be a song in this after all.

"Mr. Kaye said kidneys are their bread and butter," Miguel said.

"Makes sense," Javeed replied. "That's about eighty percent of the transplant business."

"Huh," Kristine said. "I would have assumed the need for organs would have been more equally distributed."

"You would have assumed wrong," Javeed said. "It's mostly kidneys. Livers account for about ten percent of people on the lists, hearts are only around three percent."

"I'll be damned."

"Right," Miguel said, "so I asked if kidneys were their main business would they be equipped to deal with more than that and Mr. Kaye said not to worry, that I wouldn't be the first person they had done this with." Miguel turned to aim an arched eyebrow in my direction.

"No kidding?"

"Yeah, he declined to offer any details but he assured me this wouldn't be their first eight-organ rodeo." Miguel turned to Javeed and said, "So your estimate of one to two million bucks for the entire Miguel Padilla package, was that a wild guess or was it based on something?"

"It was from a magazine article I saw a few years ago," Javeed said.

"You think the prices fluctuate?"

Javeed shrugged as Kristine pulled her phone and started a search. "I'm on it."

"Thanks," Miguel said. "I definitely want the most current information for my negotiations."

"Yeah," Javeed said, "You don't want to leave any money on the table."

At this point I went to the kitchen in search of something I could write on. I knew there was a song in all of this madness and I wanted to get it down on paper. I had decided to work with the melody from the "Battle Hymn of the Republic"; it's a good march with a nice cadence and quite rousing. I ended up having to compose the lyrics on the back of a grocery list. It was all I could find.

"OK," Kristine said. "Here's a recent article from a British science journal about the black market. It says a healthy liver can go for a hundred and sixty thousand dollars. A heart's worth close to half a million." She added the numbers for everything and said, "All totaled, it's just over a million and a half dollars."

"What did I tell you?" Javeed said.

"Does it say where the donors come from?"

"Anywhere there's poverty," Kristine said.

"My friend Mark Simmons swears the black market is alive and well and operating right here in Los Angeles," Javeed said.

"Who's Mark Simmons?"

"A cardiologist friend of mine," Javeed said. "Does lots of transplants, so he knows Jake Trapper pretty well. Mark told me a story about an elderly patient he had not long ago. This guy needed a new heart, but his age disqualified him according to SCOPE guidelines. And he was too frail to hop a twenty-three-hour flight to Egypt to get one." Javeed looked toward the ceiling as if searching for something. "What was that guy's name? Oh, Henry J. Fontaine."

"As in the billionaire Fontaines?"

"Yes indeed," Javeed said. "And, not coincidentally, the next thing Mark knew, Mr. Fontaine had a new ticker. According to his passport Fontaine hadn't been out of the country in five years, so the obvious conclusion is that it was done right here. Of course there's no way to prove Mr. Fontaine went through Mr. Kaye to get the heart, but they do have Jake Trapper in common, so…"

They spent the next few minutes vigorously speculating on where in Los Angeles you might find non-cadaver heart donors who matched your needs.

I was writing at a fever pitch now, scribbling furiously on the tiny, narrow pad of paper I had scavenged from the kitchen.

Miguel looked at me and said, "What are you doing?"

"Just keep talking," I said. "You're practically writing this song for me."

In no time at all they had concocted a thoroughly plausible scenario involving a pool of potential organ donors made up of the two million undocumented workers living in the state of California.

"You can imagine they get sick, go to a neighborhood clinic, and get some blood drawn," Javeed said. "Before you know it, there's a database with all the information you need. Then you hack in or bribe someone with access to the data and *voilà*! Organs!"

"Yes!" I said with enough verve to get their attention. "*Voilà* indeed!" I held up my newest composition and waved it like a victory flag. "This may be my best one yet. I'm not sure where it goes in the story, but this is a keeper."

"Oh, speaking of that," Miguel said. "I almost forgot. At the end of my meeting with Mr. Kaye, I told him about our project."

"What on earth for?"

"He asked what I was up to so I told him," Miguel said. "And, to my surprise, he said he knows a potential investor and—"

"What?! And you waited until now to mention this? My god, this man is dealing with billionaires on a regular basis! This could be our ticket!"

"Don't worry," Miguel said. "Mr. Kaye's going to check with the man and let me know if he's interested. Meanwhile, are you going to sing this new song or what?"

I was warming my instrument and about to start singing when the food arrived. The moment I caught the scent of turmeric, smoky cumin, and onions I abandoned all thoughts of entertaining my friends. I could practically taste the naan.

Kristine served up the chicken tikka masala over basmati rice with a side of eggplant bharta. Javeed was admiring his plate as he said, "You know, India used to be the place to go for illegal kidneys. Entire families would sell—"

"Javeed!" Kristine glared at him. "Can we not talk about carving up entire families while we eat dinner?"

"What? Oh, sure, sorry."

Kristine said grace and then we ate. And ate. And after we had scraped the last bit of dal from the container, Miguel asked again if I would sing the new song.

"Of course," I said. "You all know this one, right?" I sang: "Mine eyes have seen the glory of the coming of the Lord..." Everyone nodded their familiarity with the tune. "I'm calling this 'The Transplant Hymn of the Republic.'"

"The scene is a low-cost neighborhood clinic in Los Angeles," I said, setting the stage. "The waiting room is filled with the undocumented poor as Rich Uncle Moneybags enters from stage right pushing a shopping cart." And with that, I began to sing my heart out, so to speak.

"For half a million dollars
You can buy a pre-owned heart,
The donor has to die
But you will get a brand-new start,
So if you like your shopping
Let's get down to organ mart,
Where poor folks will provide.

Gory, gory, transplant surgery,

Black markets work just fine.

Your lungs are full of fluid
And your breaths are getting short,

You can beg for intubation
Or get down to the airport,
That man who crossed illegal
You might not want to deport,
'cause poor folks will provide.

Gory, gory, transplant surgery,

Black markets work just fine.

Let's say you need a transplant
And your budget's getting tight,
You can get yourself a cheaper one,
By hopping on a flight,
They sell kidneys, lungs, and livers
At a price that will delight,
The poor folks will provide.

Gory, gory, transplant surgery…

Gory, gory, transplant surgery…

Gory, gory, transplant surgery,

Black markets work just fine!"

***

The following Tuesday night at eight, Miguel and Javeed found themselves standing side-by-side on the second deck of an unused parking structure in Culver City, California. The scene wouldn't have been at all peculiar except for the fact that they were standing there with black bags pulled over their heads.

135

"All I'm saying is, it's possible," Javeed said.

"Of course it's possible," Miguel agreed. "Anything's possible."

"Well, not anything," Javeed argued. "It's not possible the sun will start revolving around the earth in the next ten minutes, right?"

"OK, fine," Miguel said. "It's possible this is all an elaborate scheme to get us to their facility to harvest both of us."

"That's all I'm saying," Javeed said as he adjusted his hood. "It's possible. And then what? No one will know where it happened. And it would be impossible for anyone to find out."

"Look, if we disappear," Miguel said, "the cops would eventually talk to Kristine who could tell them about Jake Trapper."

"So what?" Javeed said. "If everybody who goes to this place does it the same way we're doing it, then he wouldn't know where it happened either. So we get harvested, Mr. Kaye disappears and—"

"I'm just saying your version doesn't make much long-term sense for these guys and their business model," Miguel said. "Sure, it might be good from a quarterly earnings perspective, but then what? Why do something that would draw so much attention, you know what I mean? The goose they've got keeps laying golden eggs, why kill it?"

They stopped talking when they heard a vehicle coming up the ramp. It pulled to a stop a few yards in front of them, idling, the telltale smell of diesel wafting in the air. Then they heard a man speaking.

"Sorry about the hoods," Mr. Kaye said. "But we have to be very careful."

Javeed felt someone take his hand to shake it. "Dr. Ahmadi? I'm Mr. Kaye. Nice to meet you." One at a time he led them to the vehicle. "You'll have to step up."

Miguel had made arrangements to see the transplant facility with Javeed coming along to give a proper medical seal of approval. Once they were seated in the vehicle and buckled in, Mr. Kaye said he would start some music and that no one would talk for the duration of the trip.

It was an opera, German from the sounds of it. Miguel guessed that they drove around for the better part of an hour on both surface streets and freeways. By the time they stopped, Miguel knew they could be anywhere in any one of five counties.

The opera stopped and the doors opened. Someone helped Miguel and Javeed out of the vehicle and across a space that smelled like a garage, transmission fluid and oil. They heard elevator doors open, they were escorted inside, then the doors closed.

"You can take your hoods off if you'd like," Mr. Kaye said.

It was a standard hospital elevator, large enough for a gurney and medical personnel, wide doors on either end, all wrapped in stainless-steel cladding. They descended a floor or two before the doors opened onto a tile hallway that was buffed to an antiseptic shine.

Mr. Kaye gave them a tour, leading them down the hall past spacious rooms, some occupied, some not. Javeed thought it looked like the Four Seasons had opened a hospital. The patient rooms were first class with double-tiered headwall systems and more up-to-date equipment than Ascendant Medical.

The three operating rooms were also state of the art. There was an array of articulated overhead booms, one supporting the Seraphim robotic surgery system, others held endoscopic hardware and touch-screen displays which provided immediate access to medical records, vital signs, X-rays and MRIs.

Miguel asked Javeed what he thought. "Well," he said, "depending on who the surgeon was, I wouldn't hesitate to have a procedure done here."

"No offense," Mr. Kaye said with a smile. "But I'm not sure you could afford it on an internist's salary. We really do charge exorbitant sums for our services which, to answer your question, includes some of the best surgeons in the country."

"Yeah, how does that work?" Javeed said. "How do you get a surgeon to break the law like that? Great gobs of cash or blackmail or something else?" Javeed knew any number of surgeons who engaged in activities they would happily pay not to have exposed.

"No need for extortion," Mr. Kaye said. "As I'm sure you know, all doctors don't believe the same things, right? They don't all agree with every position the AMA takes. They don't all believe, for example, that the provision in the Anatomical Gift Act prohibiting the private sale of kidneys for transplantation is ethical, or good medicine for that matter," Mr. Kaye said. "And they don't all disagree with the AMA for the same reasons either. Some are diehard libertarians, others see it as a matter of saving more lives than the UNOS system does. Some are simply in it for the money, so yes, gobs of cash is at least part of it."

"But at the risk of losing their license?"

"Very little risk of that," Mr. Kaye said. "Everybody here works under a pseudonym. All patients and employees arrive and depart the way you did so no one can tell authorities where we are. We pay roughly three times the going rate for all service providers. We have great benefits and no one can be sued for malpractice because the patients understand there are trade-offs to getting a transplant this way."

Javeed took all of that in and said, "Listen, any chance you could use an internist?"

Mr. Kaye smiled and said, "Only if you're willing to part with a kidney."

Javeed appeared to give it some thought. "So, what's the going rate?"

"Well, I don't want to tip my hand," Mr. Kaye said, turning to Miguel. "Did you come up with a number for me?"

Miguel didn't hesitate. "I'm thinking two million," he said.

The number didn't seem to shock Mr. Kaye who replied, "Well, that's close to full retail and then only if you're AB-negative."

"Damn, Bro," Javeed said. "You're B-positive. That's rare, but not two million dollars rare."

"OK," Miguel said. "How about this…"

"I'm listening."

"If we lose the legal challenge," Miguel said, "I'll give you four organs in exchange for you transplanting the other four, at your cost, into patients who would otherwise not get them." He jerked a thumb toward Javeed. "I'm sure my friend here and Jake Trapper will be glad to find the recipients for you."

"Wait, what? I can't be involved in something like that!"

"I'd do it for you," Miguel said.

"You don't know that."

"No, but it's possible," Miguel said. "Just like your theory on why we were being brought here."

Mr. Kaye reached out and shook Miguel's hand. "We have a deal." Mr. Kaye herded them back toward the elevator. "By the way," he said, as they walked down the hallway, "the businessman I mentioned? He's very keen to meet with you about investing in your project."

"No kidding?"

"Yeah, apparently he saw the story in the paper and found the whole thing fascinating." Mr. Kaye handed Miguel a business card just as the elevator arrived. "He's expecting your call."

They stepped onto the elevator and Mr. Kaye said, "Hoods, gentlemen."

12

It was around this time that Rebecca Vaughn shared a message about our project with her seven million followers. This was excellent news for us since it put us on the radar of everyone in the industry, but it was not without its unforeseen and unintended consequences.

For Ms. Vaughn it was all about organ donation, her pet cause. She posted statistics about how many people die in the U.S. each year owing to a lack of organs (eight thousand) and how this one man, Miguel Padilla, was trying to help as many people as he could, even in his darkest hour. She also provided a link to the National Donate Life Registry as well as posting the hashtag now associated with Miguel's story: #organguy!

This was reposted hundreds of thousands of times and led to a significant, if short-lived, increase in donor registry. It was a feel-good story because, as you might expect, virtually no one is against organ donation. Ninety-five percent of Americans say they support it, (though only fifty-four percent actually register as organ donors, proving once again that talk is cheap). Still, it's safe to say organ donation is not the least bit controversial.

And if Miguel's case had only been about his desire to donate his organs, support for his cause might have been universal and no one would have come out against him.

However.

The problem was the other, inseparable, half of Miguel's case. Because even though the Right to Die movement had clear majority support across the country, it also had opponents. And a percentage of that opposition was accurately described as virulent, radical, and driven by religious fervor, which in the history of mankind has never proven to be a good combination.

And since #organguy! linked to the Lynn Mitchum interview as well as the newspaper articles about Miguel's story, it didn't just reach the organ donation crowd, it also reached those who were radically opposed to Miguel's request for physician-assisted—

No, wait. I have to stop before I use the dreaded "S" word.

(You may skip this next section if you wish, as it doesn't really move plot or character forward very much, though it will inform the motives of a few people in the story. On the other hand, if the subject of how we use language is something you find interesting, as I do, you may want to at least skim the text. I will keep this as brief as possible, so please bear with me.)

First, a little history: One of the original organizations to advocate for the right of terminally ill patients to die when and how they wanted was a group calling itself the Euthanasia Educational Council which later changed its name to Concern For Dying, which I would imagine polled much more favorably with the public given euthanasia's association with having to put down your favorite old dog and the horrors of the concentration camps.

A few years later, the cryptically named Hemlock Society was founded. They later changed their name to End-of-Life Choices which they must have agreed was more descriptive of the group's goals than naming themselves after a highly poisonous biennial herbaceous flowering plant from the carrot family. A few of that group's members later broke off to form the Final Exit Network, which, to me, sounds like a cable channel found somewhere up in the four hundreds. End-of-Life Choices later merged with a group called Compassion in Dying, which later renamed itself Compassion and Choices, which everyone agreed was a vast improvement over anything with the word euthanasia in it.

But difficult as it might be to find a suitable name for a "Right to Die" organization, imagine how much more challenging it is to give a consumer-friendly name to the act they advocate for.

My god, this has already gone on far too long so I'll try to wrap it up quickly.

Those in favor prefer terms like "Physician-assisted death" in order to avoid the emotionally fraught word "suicide." There are more flowery terms like "Death with Dignity" (which I rather like) but, if you're intent on using value-neutral language, as many of these groups insist they are, then "physician-assisted death" or "dying" is the go-to phrase.

Meanwhile, the opposition naturally insists on using the word "suicide" when talking about it because they know the word triggers heated emotions and they also know that it's easier to sway people to your position by employing emotional manipulation than it is to do so based on reason.

In any event, once Rebecca Vaughn's post about #organguy! went viral, it roused the sentiments of those violently opposed to physician-assisted death. And they began to post about it. And once it was clear how passionate people were about the issue, the trolls waded in.

Ethan Chaney had spent much of the past week tormenting sick and desperate people on the organ waiting lists but, as he would later admit in open court, he was growing bored with them. Sure, he enjoyed defacing Internet tribute sites put up by grieving families but where was the challenge in that? These people were so easily provoked into irrational, weeping rants that he decided to move on.

That's when he started reading about the whole doctor-assisted suicide thing. It blew Ethan Chaney's mind.

This was eye-opening stuff for Ethan. He had no idea this was going on right here in the U.S.A. Ethan wasn't exactly sure what radical utilitarian bioethics were, but apparently the physician-assisted suicide movement was part of the whole Deep State liberal euthanasia agenda! Ethan hadn't even known this was a thing.

Ethan was captivated by the conspiracy theories about how the doctors who were doing this were required to lie on death certificates, claiming the cause of death was some bogus underlying condition when the truth was that condition didn't actually cause the death. Just outright lie! Right on the death certificate! These people weren't really doctors, you could argue, more like "lethal prescribers" since they were just killing people with drugs. Executioners, even!

Ethan was fascinated and more than a little scared by the things he learned. This shit was rampant, but nobody was doing anything about it. In fact, more and more states were making it all legal due to the influence of Deep State operatives. According to this one guy who had written a lot of books on the subject, this was what happened when radical socialist medical ideas finally came home to roost. Damn.

It was pretty complicated if you hadn't read all the books, but, from what Ethan gathered, once you found a thread you had to follow it, see where it leads. And one of the things it leads to is money. Think about it! A lot of the killing was done simply to save money since people tend to run up big medical bills in the last months and if they "elect" to do doctor-assisted suicide, insurance companies save a ton of money. Ethan had never thought about that, but he realized it was true!

And it got worse. Infanticide was widespread! According to some of the activists who were tracking the information, babies who had minor physical or intellectual problems were routinely put down, saving billions of lifetime medical treatment. Holy Jesus!

Ethan's mind was rocked when he came across a unifying theory that suggested a big part of the whole physician-assisted suicide thing was all about getting organs for the elites. It made sense, when you thought about it. They're not going to get in line like the hoi polloi and hope they get a heart or a lung or whatever. And Ethan saw the charts and grafts that proved it. This was unreal!

Ethan Chaney had found a new calling. He had to do more research, find out what was going on, and who was behind it. He decided to get involved. He started by creating a new hashtag for Miguel Padilla's story: #cultureofdeathguy!

It would soon be trending.

***

The next day, the California Superior Court notified Kristine there would be a hearing to allow the State to address the questions raised in her filing: "The State is ordered to show cause why the request for immediate declaratory relief should not be granted."

As you can imagine, this was a thrilling turn of events for us. Lives hanging in the balance and all of that. I wanted to be there for moral support and of course to make detailed notes for the inevitable courtroom scenes I would write.

I had envisioned the case taking place downtown, in a courthouse with an imposing classical Roman temple form, but we ended up in Chatsworth at a somewhat more prosaic structure. In fact, owing to the remodeling of two floors of the actual courthouse, we found ourselves in one of several repurposed mobile homes situated in the parking lot, a perfectly suitable setting for fighting a traffic ticket, perhaps, but a rather dispiriting venue for a monumental battle over constitutional rights. But there we were.

Javeed took the day off to join me in the gallery in support of his friend.

Now, anyone who isn't clever enough to dodge jury duty knows that hearings and trials do not unfold like taut television dramas. There are formalities and delays and paperwork. In fact it is so deathly boring I'm surprised more defendants don't just strike a plea bargain in order to end the misery of it all or at least demand that the time wasted be subtracted from their eventual sentence.

My point being that instead of subjecting you to the mind-numbing minutiae we suffered through, I will focus your attention on the highlights of the hearing. And while it's possible I might miss a few legal particulars, I think you will agree that the trade-off is worthwhile.

In any event, after slogging through some procedural matters it was agreed that both sides would refer to the two laws in question as AB-15 and UAGA instead of by their more unwieldy names, The End of Life Option Act and the Uniform Anatomical Gift Act. That bit of business having been dealt with, we finally reached the moment for opening statements.

The State, apparently already bored by the proceedings, bolted from the gate by making a motion to immediately dismiss on the grounds that the plaintiff had failed to state a claim for which relief could be granted.

The judge asked for Kristine's thoughts on that.

"As we stated in our documents, Your Honor," she said, "relief is easily granted by allowing an exemption to the wording of AB-15. My client should not be denied his right to donate his organs simply because the legislature failed to anticipate a circumstance as unusual as the one in front of the court."

Kristine went on to argue that there were three parts of the law that were the cause of the problem, all of which were easily fixed. First was the requirement that the physician-assisted death could not occur "in a public place", which meant it couldn't be done in a hospital.

"Under normal circumstances, this makes perfect sense," Kristine said. "But these are not normal circumstances."

Kristine went on to say that Miguel being forced to die in a non-public place (meaning at home) made it unreasonably difficult to exercise his right to donate his organs since most homes are not equipped with a sterile surgical suite.

"Furthermore," she said, "while the requirement that the means of death be a dose of barbiturates makes perfect sense in the vast majority of cases where the patient had no desire to donate their organs, here such a requirement interferes with my client's desire to exercise his rights under UAGA."

The State rose to say, "Your Honor, even if we allowed an exemption for these points, the law, in order to remove any taint of homicide, requires the patient to self-administer the… the thing that will lead to death and since Mr. Padilla is asking—"

"Let me save you the time of finishing your thought," Kristine interrupted. "Since it seems obvious that one cannot remove one's own organs, that is why we seek an exemption in the self-administering clause of AB-15."

The judge said, "Might I ask who would be doing this surgery since it won't be Mr. Padilla himself? Wouldn't a surgeon be violating some aspect of his or her licensing requirements?"

"Your Honor," Kristine said. "All that need be done is for the court to stipulate that this particular act, in this particular circumstance, is neither surgery nor the practice of medicine."

"How's that?"

"Surgery is the treatment of injuries or disorders of the body by incision or manipulation, especially with instruments," Kristine said. "Simply removing organs does not meet that definition, thus it isn't surgery. It is not being done to heal Mr. Padilla; there is no surgery that can heal him. Nor could it reasonably be considered the practice of medicine since again it is not intended to treat a malady." Kristine went on to explain how the legislators in the great State of Georgia had arranged their workaround on lethal executions with similar verbal legerdemain.

At this point there was a sidebar, followed by some more paperwork, and a fifteen-minute recess. I went in search of a restroom and a decent cup of coffee which took far longer than expected. When I returned, the hearing was back in full swing and had taken a turn away from the language of AB-15.

Kristine was saying, "In Washington v. Glucksberg, the Ninth Circuit affirmed that a citizen's right to die was a fundamental liberty interest protected by the Due Process Clause and therefor—"

"Yes," the State interjected. "But the Supreme Court overturned the Ninth Circuit on Glucksberg."

"Yes they did," Kristine acknowledged. "But they did so only because at the time it wasn't a right that was, and I quote, deeply rooted in U.S. history and tradition and implicit in the concept of ordered liberty, end quote."

"So?"

"So, twenty-four years ago when Glucksberg was in front of the court, the right-to-die movement was only twenty years old. If we take the Karen Anne Quinlan case as the beginning of the move toward right-to-die legislation, that puts us nearly forty years later today," Kristine said. "And only someone in need of a corneal transplant can't see that the law is going to continue evolving in this direction. Like women's rights and civil rights, the change is slow in coming and it is incremental, but it is undeniably moving forward."

Kristine continued by saying, "Since 1994, nine states in the U.S. have passed legislation legalizing physician-assisted dying or had it implemented by court order. So my question is: When does something finally become deeply rooted in U.S. history and tradition and implicit in the concept of ordered liberty? Is it after fifty years? A hundred? A thousand?"

"Perhaps it's like pornography," the State said. "We will know it when we see it, but until then…"

The judge gave the State a mild rebuke for the flippancy of the comment and then said to Kristine, "Your point is well taken and it's an excellent question. Unfortunately this court does not have the answer to it."

The State then raised a procedural issue of some sort which triggered a lengthy back-and-forth between all parties, quite dense and so tedious that I drifted off. When I woke, the State was still going on about the Glucksberg affair.

"The court found that the ban on physician-assisted dying was rationally related to the state's interest in, above all, the protection of human life," the State said.

Kristine jumped her feet. "Protection of human life? Your Honor, it occurs to me that this is all just a variation on the trolley problem."

In case you missed it in college, the trolley problem is an old thought exercise involving a runaway trolley. Ahead, on the tracks, there are five people tied up and unable to move. The trolley is headed straight for them. You are standing some distance off in the train yard, next to a lever. If you pull this lever, the trolley will switch to a different set of tracks. However, you notice there is one person on the side track. You have two options: Do nothing and allow the trolley to kill the five people on the main track or pull the lever, diverting the trolley onto the side track where it will kill but one person.

"But with eight people on the tracks instead of five," the Judge said. "That number was arbitrary anyway, right? It just needed to be more than one to make the problem interesting."

"More importantly," Kristine said, "the one person on the other track in our case has two terminal diseases. You're killing someone who is about to die and who in a sound state of mind has put himself on the track intentionally."

"All true and interesting," the judge said. "However since the trolley problem has never been adjudicated, it gives us no precedent on which to rely, no guidance to help steer our course."

"Of course, I just suddenly noticed the parallel," Kristine said. "So back to the State's interest in, above all, the protection of human life... What is the legitimate State interest in allowing eight people to die when their deaths can be prevented simply by allowing the exceptions to the language we have discussed so that my client can exercise all of his rights?"

"Your Honor," the State said. "It's an incomplete hypothetical and calls for speculation."

"OK," the judge said. "But out of curiosity, if the State's interest is in, above all, the protection of human life, can you tell us why the State would sacrifice the lives of eight people to prevent one from exercising his rights in an atypical fashion?"

"The State is not here to answer theoretical questions, Your Honor."

"That's what I thought."

The State then said, "The statute was written by the legislature and if Mr. Padilla wants to change the statute, he must get the legislature to do so."

Kristine pointed out that Miguel was dying and so lacked the time required to lobby the California State Assembly which is why they were seeking immediate relief in the first place, but the argument fell on deaf ears.

Kristine then returned to her Bi-Metallic Investment Company v. State Board of Equalization argument about how due process applied when the State acted against an individual. And how, when the State did so, the court had to review the matter, taking into consideration the unique individual circumstances of the case.

"And in the case of Miguel Padilla," Kristine said, "that means the court must ask if the unique characteristics presented by his circumstance warrants immediate declaratory relief. Which we assert it does."

The State countered with an argument so convoluted and tone deaf that it hit my ears like an entire side of a Yoko Ono record. I tried to follow the caterwauling but could make neither head nor tails of the point the State was trying to make. But it ended with, "In other words, Your Honor, there must be a limit to individual argument in such matters if government is to go on."

149

"Look," Kristine said. "All the State has to do is acknowledge that Mr. Padilla has the right to both donate his organs and to die with dignity. And all they have to do for this to happen is make an exemption in AB-15, and allow his organ donation to be his means of dying."

At this point the State clutched its pearls and said it was frightfully worried about the old slippery slope.

To which Kristine replied, "You're saying the State is afraid that if it allows Mr. Padilla to do this, the citizens of the state of California will be lining up en masse to be harvested to death?"

"We dare not take the chance," the State said, somehow maintaining a serious expression.

"I think we've heard enough," the judge said. "The court will consider your positions and will issue a ruling as soon as possible." She banged her gavel and sent us packing.

***

The next afternoon Kristine called each of us to say she had received an email from the court. It was a punch to the gut. They had rejected our request for relief.

I knew this was going to be a hard blow for everyone, but at least now I could write the courtroom scene, moving the script one step closer to completion. This would be the low point of the story, of course—the big gloom, some call it—where a round defeat leaves our hero in despair that he may never reach his goal.

This would unquestionably be in the play because a play needs moments like this. And moments like this need a song, something with lyrics that were sorrowful without being depressing and angry without being wrathful. It needed to say people were dying and we need someone with the courage to step up and do something about it. And, if it could be done without undermining the righteousness of the wounded, it needed just the slightest hint of assigning blame. All of these conditions seemed to call out for an old spiritual or a hymn perhaps. Perhaps "We Shall Overcome?" But no, it's too repetitive.

I had a few hours to kill, so I sat down and got to work on it.

We met that night at ICU to commiserate and drown our sorrows. I had finished the song and had it in my pocket. It was a thing of beauty written to the tune of "Will the Circle Be Unbroken," and it accomplished exactly what I needed it to. I hoped the right moment would present itself tonight, so I could sing it for them.

"The ruling was pretty bare bones," Kristine said. "AB-15 and UAGA are considered legal rights, not constitutional rights. And since both laws are clearly constitutional on their own, they're subject only to a rational basis test which the laws easily pass."

"But what about the unique circumstance angle?"

"They punted on that," Kristine said. "The court simply didn't want to go there. It was too messy. They said you were free to exercise your right to AB-15. They also said the State wasn't preventing you from exercising your rights under UAGA. They said the brain tumor and the ALS were doing that, not the State."

"Damn," Javeed said. "Tricky bastards."

"So that's it?"

"I'm afraid so," Kristine said. "We tried, but it's all over. Case closed."

"Just like that?" Miguel didn't want to hear it. "We can't quit now!"

"I'm sorry, Miguel, I really am," Kristine said. "I may have overreached. I shouldn't have gotten your hopes up." She squeezed his hand.

"You have to admit, it was a pretty big ask," Javeed said.

"Wait, what about the class action angle? The medical self-defense thing. I'm starting to like that one," Miguel said. "Can't you file another suit?"

"Not unless we can find another claim," Kristine said. "They closed the door. That was our one bite at that apple."

Javeed draped his arm over Miguel's shoulder. "I'm sorry, buddy. I guess we got a little caught up in the moment."

"But…"

"You have to let it go," Javeed said. "We set the bar too high, that's all."

We looked at one another, sadness mixed with pride from having given it the old college try.

"But, hey," Kristine said, "We gave it a good shot, didn't we?"

Miguel looked at us, fondly, and said, "I can still save one life though, right, if I donate a kidney?"

Javeed nodded. "Or more than that if you decide to go with Mr. Kaye's locally sourced, small-batch organ-removal and artisanal transplant service," he said.

Miguel laughed. "I suppose I need to consider that now. I mean if it saves eight lives, it shouldn't matter that some of them are rich."

"Yes, no point in holding that against the poor bastards," I said. "And what a thing that would be, saving lives, even rich lives."

"So it's still a win," Miguel said. "Just not the one we were hoping for."

"Are you kidding? It's a huge win," Javeed said. "And you will be remembered for it."

Miguel motioned to the waitress for another round of drinks. "Thanks for trying, Kristine. You did great," he said. "The law failed us, but you didn't." He leaned over and kissed her cheek. "I knew I could count on you, all of you. I just hope you know how much I love you guys."

At this point I felt things tipping uncomfortably toward the maudlin, and felt I needed to do something to lift the mood at the table so I reached over and touched Miguel saying, "Listen, I'm very

sorry about the court's finding but… you're still going to die, right?"
I let that land before I broke into a smile.

Miguel smiled as well. "Yeah, I'm pretty sure about that."

"Good, because you know, otherwise… it screws up the ending."

"I wouldn't do that to you," Miguel said. "The show must go on!"

13

The next round of drinks arrived and Miguel raised his glass, giving a nod to Javeed and Kristine who understood his meaning while leaving me out in the cold. Once again they declared, "*Lex clavatoris designati rescindenda est!*" And again they tipped their glasses to drink like victorious gladiators.

"What on earth *is* that?" I said.

"Latin," Javeed replied.

I gave him a wounded look. "*Et tu, Brute?*" I said, having suddenly remembered one more phrase in the language.

Kristine laughed and said, "The three of us were our own little fraternity back in college. That's our secret motto."

"What does it mean?"

Javeed said, "What does 'secret' mean?"

"I vote we tell him," Miguel said. "Maybe he can put it in the play."

"Fine with me," Kristine said, raising her hand.

Javeed shrugged and lifted his hand as well, saying, "Yeah, I'm good with that."

Miguel beckoned me to approach, as though preparing to reveal an ancient and mystical secret. I leaned closer as he glanced about to see if anyone could hear him before he said, "*Lex clavatoris designati rescindenda est* means... The designated hitter rule has to go!"

"It's an abomination!" Kristine said, rather loudly.

"Makes a mockery of the game." Javeed waved a hand like swatting at a fly.

To their eternal surprise I thumped my fist on the table proudly and said, "You will be pleased to know I've been saying that since 1973, though in English."

"Get out!" Kristine said.

"No," I said. "Honestly, it rewards one-dimensional players and cheapens the sport I have loved since I was a young boy attending games at the Polo Grounds."

So thrilled were they at this unexpected revelation, my three friends cheered! I felt this was my d'Artagnan moment, me joining the formidable Musketeers of the Guard at long last. And we raised our glasses again and we drank.

Then we ordered more drinks and proceeded to get quite drunk. After the next round it was fair to say Javeed was very nearly embalmed. He slapped his palm on the table and said, "You know what? Screw Mr. Kaye! I'll do it."

"Do what?" Miguel said.

"I'll harvest you!" Javeed giggled.

Kristine rolled her eyes and said, "We discussed this earlier, Javeed, remember? Homicide, prison, all that?"

"I'll spatchcock your ass!" Javeed giggled again. "And I'll give all the parts to the poor, just the way you want!"

"Well, don't call me to defend you," Kristine said. "I'm strictly wills and trusts from here on."

"I'll defend myself," Javeed said. "Anyway, that's not the point. The point is my friend asked me to do something for him and I intend to do it. It'll be great! We'll drape your living room with plastic or something and I'll get some rib spreaders from somewhere and grab a carving knife and boom! We'll do it. It'll be great!"

Miguel played along, saying, "You'd risk your reputation for me? Your freedom? Your whole future?"

"For you? Hell yes, I would," Javeed said.

"You'd… kill me?"

"I'd love to!"

They laughed and hugged each other the way two happy drunks will do.

I was thrilled. "This is fantastic!" That entertaining bit of inebrious dialogue had given me an idea. "What a wonderful scene this will be!" I went to the bar to get pen and paper so I could jot some notes lest I forget the idea in the wake of my own considerable intoxication. I scribbled some words and stuffed the paper in the pocket where I felt the new song waiting patiently for its debut.

It was getting late now and I felt the mood was right. We were the last table in the restaurant. I pulled the new song from my pocket and showed it to Miguel who I asked to join on the chorus and for the verse I'd written for him to sing. I asked Kristine and Javeed to hum the melody as accompaniment. And once we settled on a tempo, I began to sing.

"They've been waiting, on the list, lord,

Many cold and cloudy days,

They don't want that hearse a-comin',

For to carry them away."

The wait staff noticed and began drifting in our direction as Miguel and I sang the chorus.

"Well the list keeps getting longer,

For the young child and the old,

There are ways to make it shorter,

But the courts just ain't that bold."

Again, I soloed, the wait staff entranced.

"Some object to giving money,

To the donors who provide,

They say it exploits those who need cash,

And the dying are just brushed aside."

Kristine joined us this time.

"Well the list keeps getting longer,
For the young child and the old,
There are ways to make it shorter,
But politicians just ain't that bold."
Miguel's verse.
"I was trying to help others,
When the state said, no you don't.
We have rules and regulations,
To help make sure that you won't."
Javeed and two of the waiters joined for the final chorus,
"Well the list keeps getting longer,
For the young child and the old,
There are ways to make it shorter,
But none seem to be that bold…"
The alcohol had inflicted its maudlin effects onto several of us, and we dabbed the tears from our eyes when the song was over. The wait staff, which we assumed had come over expressly to join us in song and marvel at our voices, had in fact come to take our car keys from us.

We agreed that was a capital idea and Kristine arranged for a ride-sharing service to collect us. After settling our bill, we piled into an SUV while singing at the top of our lungs.

"Does the tissue match?
That's the one big catch!
Blood types matter, you can bet your ass,
Get on your knees and pray."
This was followed by gales of laughter and discussions about which song to sing next.

The driver, a handsome young man from another country, seemed thoroughly charmed by our song and asked what it was all about. We explained Miguel's situation and said the court had rejected our request but (and here, I can only blame the liquor) we told him we knew about an underground hospital where they would remove all of Miguel's organs for transplant, so the problem had been sorted.

This didn't seem to faze the driver in the slightest. In fact, he seemed quite keen to know more.

Realizing I had said too much already, I redirected the conversation. "In any event," I said, "we have taken this unfortunate situation and we're going to produce an opera!"

"I have never understood opera," the driver said. "They are never in my language."

"Well, this is more like a musical," I said. "And it's in English, so…"

"Like this one," Miguel said before he began to belt this one out:

"Let's say you need a transplant,
But your budget's getting tight."
The rest of us joined in, lustily.
"You can get yourself a cheaper one
By hopping on a flight.
They sell kidneys, lungs, and livers
At a price that will delight.
The poor folks will provide!"
The driver eyed us in the mirror as we hooted and cackled and tried to catch our breath.

When we finally settled down, the driver said, "I would sell one of my kidneys for the right price." He looked over his shoulder at me. "How much will they give me at this hospital?"

This was a rather sobering thing to hear, but it wasn't enough to make me clear-headed. I said, "My good man, we don't, uh, I don't, uh, you misunderstood."

"I want to go to college but the tuition, it is insane," the driver said. "I have three jobs and I can barely afford my rent."

I knew I had to nip this in the bud. "I understand," I said. "Why don't you give me your number and I will pass it on to the right people." I looked at him seriously as if I actually meant it.

The driver pulled a card from the visor and handed it to me. "That is my cell. Call me any time," he said. "I am serious. I want to get a degree."

"I understand and that's most admirable." I said. "But I can't make any promises."

Quite out of the blue, and serving as an excellent distraction, Kristine began to recite the Declaration of Independence.

"We hold these toothes to be self-evident," she slurred. "Not toothes, truths! And that all men are endowed by their Creator…" She nudged me with her elbow and said, "Though to tell you the truth, some men are more endowed than others." Then she winked.

"Excuse me," the driver said. "You left out the part that all men are created equal."

"What? Oh, yes, you're right." Kristine said. "Thank you. And are endowed by their Creator with certain unin… uninsalable… unintentional…"

"Unalienable," I said.

Kristine clapped a hand onto my leg and said, "Yes! Thank you. Unalienable, whew, that's a tough one! Unalienable rights and among these are Life, Liberty, and the pursuit of Happiness," she said. "So I gotta ask, how much liberty do you really have if you can't donate all your organs whenever you want to? Huh? You call that freedom? Don't tread on me!" She turned to look at Javeed. "Did you know that the original words were Life, Liberty, and…"

She stopped, looking somewhat stricken. I couldn't tell if she had had a sudden revelation or if she was about to be sick.

"Should we pull to the side of the road?"

"I don't believe it," she said. "It's properly, no, property! That's it."

"Life, liberty, and property? Yes, I believe that's the original phrase," I said. "What of it?"

Kristine leaned close to me, rested her head on my shoulder, said, "Property," and then she began to snore.

***

It took some doing, but by the time we reached Kristine's house we had managed to wake her enough that we didn't have to carry her inside. We escorted her in a corkscrew fashion up the walkway to the door where she assured us she would be fine and said we should all meet at Miguel's in the morning to get to work on the lawsuit.

Confused, Miguel said, "We already lost the lawsuit."

"Exactly." Kristine closed the door behind her, then opened it again, just slightly. She peeked out the crack and said, "We're gonna sue the bastards again." And with that she closed the door in our faces and threw the bolt.

We returned to our ride agreeing that Kristine's comment about a new lawsuit was the result of her general state of fustication, but agreed to meet at Miguel's anyway for a hangover brunch and some hair of the dog.

Late the next morning, after liberating our cars from ICU parking lot, Javeed and I stopped at a local eatery famous for its corned beef hash and fried potatoes. We bought enough for a platoon and arrived at Miguel's around eleven, where we immediately made a pitcher of Bloody Marys to help ease our pain.

Kristine arrived behind a pair of dark glasses about twenty minutes later. The first thing she saw when she walked into the room was me, bent over a kitchen stool with my trousers pulled down as Javeed approached from behind.

Kristine staggered to a stop and said, "Whoa!", peering over the shades for clarification.

Javeed plunged a hypodermic into my gluteus. "B12 shot," Javeed said.

"Thank god."

"What did you think?"

"Never mind that."

Javeed held up the syringe and said, "You want one?"

"Not if I have to drop my trousers."

"No," Javeed said. "Your arm's fine."

"What?" I stood indignantly, fixing my trousers. "You told me—"

Javeed smiled. "Just having some fun," he said.

Kristine opted for both a Bloody Mary and a shot of B12. Miguel plated the food and we dove in headfirst, as was our custom.

"So," Kristine said, "why are we here?"

"You're the one who called the meeting," Javeed said.

"Me? Why?"

"You said we were going to sue the bastards again," I said.

"Really." Kristine had no idea. "Did I say why, or how, or on what grounds?"

"Something to do with the Declaration of Independence bit about life, liberty, and property," I said. "You seemed less concerned with life and liberty than you were about the property part.'"

Kristine shoveled a forkful of potatoes into her mouth and tried to remember. She chewed for a moment before she covered her mouth and said, "Oh my god, that's right. I remember now. I had some kind of a property argument." She finished chewing, swallowed, and said, "But now I don't remember what it was."

"You were thinking it was a lawsuit last night," Javeed said.

"Yeah, well, I was pretty drunk," Kristine said.

"Yes, it's fair to say we were all tight as boiled owls," I said. "But you seemed to think you were onto something useful."

"Maybe I was," Kristine said. "But it's currently lost in the folds of my throbbing brain. I mean, I know there have been cases about the application of property law to body parts but I must have seen a new angle last night, or thought I had, but I'm way too hungover to think about it at the moment."

"Maybe if you drink some more you can find it again," Miguel said.

"I suppose that might work." Kristine looked at her Bloody Mary and said, "But it's probably better if I just do some research instead. Oh, what the hell, a little bit of both." She took a drink and turned to look in my direction. "Speaking of drunk, Leonard, did you tell our driver last night about the underground hospital and the illegal surgery thing?"

"I'm afraid so," I admitted. "But I can't see any harm coming from that. In the first place the young man said he wanted to sell a kidney himself. Secondly, let's say he went to the police for some reason. Hard to imagine they're going to launch an investigation into an alleged secret underground transplant hospital based on secondhand information provided by four cross-eyed drunks."

"OK," Miguel said. "So, Kristine, you'll be researching the property thing while Leonard and I try to get a meeting with our potential investor."

"Yes, and what exactly do we know about this gentleman?" I asked.

"Dr. Steven Brewer founded The Medicus Group," Javeed said. "I read somewhere that he's got a net worth in the neighborhood of $500 million."

"Holy crowbar," Kristine said. "What is he, like a combination brain and heart surgeon?"

"As a matter of fact, and court record," Javeed said, "he was one of the worst general practitioners ever to set foot in a doctor's office. Famous for having graduated near the bottom of his class at a medical school—and I use that term loosely—located somewhere in the Lesser Antilles, Dr. Brewer somehow managed to pass the boards and get a job in a low-income neighborhood clinic where he misdiagnosed an aortic dissection as gas, may the patient rest in peace," Javeed said. "That and a couple of other championship-level bouts of malpractice led him to surrender his license without having to admit or deny anything."

"And then what?" Kristine said. "Somebody gave him half a billion dollars?"

"No, then he opened a medical supply store," Javeed said. "You know, bedpans, walkers, stool softeners, that sort of thing. It was such a success that he opened several more around the state, then expanded throughout the Southwest. Meanwhile he moved into the wholesale hospital supply business. Then he bought a couple of non-emergency medical transport companies and merged them into the largest outfit in Southern California. If the guy had a press, he couldn't print money any faster."

"I like the sounds of this one," I said.

"Me too," Kristine said. "Is he single?"

"I'll be sure to ask," Miguel said.

***

I was with Miguel two days later when he had another seizure. We were standing in his kitchen talking about the new scene and going over the song I had written for our pitch to Dr. Brewer.

One moment all was well, then an unsettled look crossed Miguel's face and it seemed as if he knew what was coming. I had no idea what was happening at the time. I just noticed an odd change in his manner. Miguel reached awkwardly for one of the stools and managed to seat himself before the cancer gripped him in ungodly pain.

He made an awful guttural noise as he placed his hands on either side of his head, lowering it to the counter. It's a terrible thing to watch someone suffer so and be unable to help in the slightest way. I remembered Javeed saying there was nothing to be done when this happened but knowing that didn't quiet the instinct to help; it simply heightened my feeling of helplessness.

The seizure didn't last twenty seconds, but it seemed like an eternity. I placed my hand on Miguel's back and asked if there was something I could do. Miguel slowly shook his head but didn't speak. I feebly poured a glass of water for him and urged him to relax.

"I'll call to cancel with Dr. Brewer," I said.

"Don't," Miguel said. "I'll be OK."

Within ten minutes he seemed better and insisted he was fine to do the pitch meeting. I could see the seizure had drained him, but he wasn't going to cancel. So we went.

The drive to Beverly Hills would take forty minutes. On the way I kept checking on Miguel out of the corner of my eye until he said, "Would you stop that? I'm fine."

"How do you do it?" I asked. "How do you get up every day and carry on in such a cheerful way, like the worst thing that could happen is that we flub the pitch?"

"What else should I do? I'm going to die and there's nothing I can do to stop that," Miguel said. "Being morose isn't any fun. Being irritable wastes a lot of energy and pushes people away. I might as well be cheerful on my way out, don't you think?"

"It's not that I disagree," I said. "I just don't know how you do it. I certainly couldn't."

We drove in silence for a moment before Miguel said, "It was my mom. She died of cancer about ten years ago. She was in pain a lot of the time but she rarely showed it. She wanted me to be proud of how she handled herself. She would tell me her death was the continuation of her great adventure, of which I was a part, and that the best way forward was with a sense of curiosity and fearlessness," he said. "I guess I learned it from her."

"So you're not frightened at all?"

"Oh no, I'm plenty scared," Miguel said. "But I refuse to just curl up and wait for the Grim Reaper. That's no way to go. The thing is, fear doesn't stop death so much as it stops life, in the same way worry doesn't take away tomorrow's problems so much as it takes away today's peace."

"That's a lovely way to look at it."

"I think I saw that on a motivational calendar," Miguel said. "But I think it's true. Anyway, another thing mom taught me was that the secret to happiness is having something to look forward to. And, right now, I'm looking forward to this play being staged."

At that moment I couldn't have loved Miguel more if he had been my own son.

14

Dr. Brewer's office was on the top floor of a new building on Wilshire Boulevard. While Javeed had been accurate in his description of The Medicus Group and its holdings, there was one part of the business of which he was unaware.

It turned out that after establishing the Medicus brand in the traditional fields of the medical supply industry, Dr. Brewer was in exactly the right place at the right time to move into the medical cannabis business. A few years later, when California legalized recreational use, he expanded his already substantial empire.

Dr. Brewer was now the proud owner of a dozen dispensaries and a grow site that supplied them. Unfortunately, due to the Federal nature of the U.S. banking system, he had the ongoing problem of finding places to park enormous sums of cash. This caused him a great deal of anxiety and sleepless nights until he discovered the calming effects of THC-infused gummies. He kept a crystal bowl filled with them on his desk.

Dr. Brewer welcomed us into his spacious office, offering coffee and pastries. He had a calm, slightly glazed look about him. "Mr. Padilla, I'm at a loss for what to say about your medical situation," he said. "But you have both my sympathy and admiration for..."

Dr. Brewer seemed to lose his train of thought, so I said, "... sympathy and admiration for... what Miguel is trying to do?"

"Hmm? Oh, yes," Dr. Brewer said. "That's it."

"Thanks very much, Dr. Brewer, and please call me Miguel."

"When I read the story in the *Times*, I was fascinated," Dr. Brewer said. "And when my friend Mr. Kaye told me about your project, well, I knew..."

Dr. Brewer glanced out the window as if he'd seen a squirrel or something. I said, "That's when you knew... you wanted to be involved in the project?"

"Hmm? Yes, that's right, exactly," Dr. Brewer said. "I would love to."

"Have you invested in theatre previously?" I asked.

"No, I haven't," Dr. Brewer said. "I hope that isn't disqualifying."

"Heavens no, not in the least," I said. "But before we talk about business, let me give you a sense of what we have in mind from the creative side."

"Oh please do," Dr. Brewer said.

I launched into the pitch, getting through the first act to where I'm introduced, giving him bits of the songs and explaining the drama of the faces on the TV screens peering down at the action as the countdown clocks ratchet up the tension.

"Then," I said, "after the court rejects their suit, a sense of gloom and defeat settles over our players. They see no way forward and they prepare to accept the loss, when, from out of nowhere, Miguel's friend, the doctor, says he will do the harvest himself. Blackout! End of scene."

Dr. Brewer was mesmerized or possibly just deeply stoned. Either way was fine as far as I was concerned. He plucked a bright-red gummy from the bowl on his desk and popped it into his mouth, sucking on it as I continued.

"The next scene opens at Miguel's apartment, now completely draped in white sheets," I said. "The doctor, Javeed, is at the door accepting a delivery from an unseen person as the producer, that's me, and the lawyer, Kristine, are perched on stools and step-ladders, poised to put up the final sheet which will cover the front door. Miguel is nowhere to be seen.

"Closing the door behind him, Javeed rolls into the apartment a stainless-steel machine about the size of a large outdoor grill and conspicuously marked with the famous logo of The Medicus Group. He rolls it to the middle of the room and proclaims, 'Thank god for Amazon Prime!'

"Kristine says, 'Is that a heart-lung machine?'

"'Yes,' Javeed replies. 'And delivered in under two hours! God, I love this country.'

"Kristine asks if the doctor knows how to operate the machine.

"'Me?' Javeed replies. 'If I'm working the bypass, who's doing the harvest? Poke around on the Internet,' he says, 'see if you can find a how-to video.'

"Kristine agrees to do this but says, 'What if I do it wrong and he... dies?'

"Everyone turns slowly to look at her.

"'Oh,' she says. 'Right. Forget I said anything.'

"Javeed tosses a package to Kristine and Leonard and says, 'Here, put these scrubs on.'

"While Kristine and Leonard disappear behind the sheets to change, Javeed plugs in the heart-lung machine and fiddles with the buttons. When he's satisfied, he looks around the room and says, 'Where's Miguel?'"

KRISTINE (*off stage*)   He went to change. Said he'd be right back.

(JAVEED *pulls a standard angle grinder from one of the packages. He calls to the back of the apartment*)

JAVEED   Miguel? You OK?

(LEONARD *enters from behind the sheets, wearing surgical scrubs, snapping his fingers and singing to the tune of "Ain't We Got Fun?"*)

LEONARD   Every morning,
                     Every evening,
                     Ain't you got parts?

(MIGUEL *enters from stage left in a hospital gown,*
fingers snapping. He joins LEONARD)

MIGUEL   Graft survival,
                     There's no rival,
                     Here, take my heart!

LEONARD   My kidney's failing.
                     Man I'm ailing…
                     The pain's off the chart.

MIGUEL   Cyclosporin,
                     There's no ignoring,
                     It's the state of the art…

LEONARD   It stops rejection,
                     There's no infection,
                     So just take me apart!

(*The two of them fall into a fit of laughter and embrace one another*)

MIGUEL   I really like that one, but it still needs a
                     few verses.

LEONARD   I'm afraid it needs more than that,
                     actually. But I think it's a keeper.

(JAVEED *comes over and checks* MIGUEL's *eyes*)

JAVEED   Are you stoned?

MIGUEL   Are you kidding? I'm higher than a
                 mountain goat! Vaped an eighth of some
                 serious blue-green kush and I'm feeling
                 noooo pain. Nada! Dadadada. But I am a
                 little hungry.

JAVEED   So you want to skip the general
                 anesthesia?

            (JAVEED *revs the angle grinder*)

MIGUEL   I never said that! I'll take whatever you've
                 got.

    (JAVEED *leans down behind the sofa and props up a large cylinder
                    tank of gas*)

JAVEED   Don't worry, I got you covered.

    (KRISTINE *enters from behind the sheets wearing scrubs and surgical
              cap. She has a document in hand*)

KRISTINE   Miguel, you never signed your will.

    (*Another one of the countdown clocks reaches 00:00. The face on
    the screen fades out, only to be replaced by a new face and a new
                    countdown clock*)

MIGUEL   Wait, I never told you who gets my
                 estate.

KRISTINE   Oh, right. I'll add that. What did you
                 decide?

MIGUEL   It all goes to the two people who were
                      there for me when I needed them
                      most. You and Javeed, right? I mean, who
                      else?

(KRISTINE *hugs* MIGUEL, *who signs the will. The two then
move the coffee table aside while* LEONARD *and* JAVEED *move
the dining table to the center of the room. They drape a sheet over it.
They take the shade off the standing lamp, tie a rope to the bottom,
toss the rope over a rafter and hoist the lamp upside down so it acts as
overhead surgical lamp*)

JAVEED   I think we're about ready.

(JAVEED *pats the "operating table,"*
MIGUEL *hops up on the table, legs swinging*)

MIGUEL   By the way, I assume you know what
                      you're doing?

JAVEED   For god's sake, I did an eight-week
                      surgery rotation at one of the finest
                      medical schools in the state where,
                      you may recall, we were fraternity
                      brothers!

MIGUEL   Yes! G.D.I. till the day I die... which I
                      guess is today!

JAVEED / MIGUEL / KRISTINE
                      Lex clavatoris designati rescindenda est!

LEONARD   What on earth was that?

KRISTINE	The three of us had our own little fraternity back in college. That's our secret motto.
LEONARD	What does it mean?
MIGUEL	You mind if I tell him? I'd rather not take that one to the grave.
JAVEED	Fine with me.
KRISTINE	Yeah, who cares?

(MIGUEL *beckons* LEONARD *to approach*)

MIGUEL	Lex clavatoris designati rescindenda est means… The designated hitter rule has to go!
JAVEED / KRISTINE	Amen!

(*The three of them high five and fist bump before* JAVEED *snaps on his surgical gloves*)

JAVEED	Alright, I think we're all set.
LEONARD	How is this going to work?
JAVEED	After we knock him out, we'll put him on bypass so we can get the heart-lung bloc out the door. Meanwhile, the other organs are still getting oxygenated blood.

LEONARD   Is that how it's normally done?

JAVEED   Does any part of this strike you as
                     normal?

(LEONARD *shakes his head as* JAVEED *puts on safety
goggles and revs the angle grinder*)

JAVEED (*To* KRISTINE)

                     OK, when I get the chest cracked,
                     text that number I gave you. By the time
                     I get the heart and lungs out, they'll be at
                     the window waiting for it.

(JAVEED *looks at everybody*)

JAVEED   Are we ready?

KRISTINE   Wait!

(KRISTINE *tenderly touches* MIGUEL's *face*)

KRISTINE   Greater love hath no man than this;
                     that a man lay down his life for others.
                     Miguel, you are the most amazing
                     person I've ever known. What you're
                     doing is... well, you're my hero. I'll
                     always love you and I'll pray for you
                     and make sure you're not forgotten.
                     Goodbye.

(*They hug*)

JAVEED   OK, are we ready now?

(*Everybody gives a thumbs-up.* JAVEED *puts a hand to* MIGUEL's
cheek, gives him a loving pat)

JAVEED   Miguel, I love you too. You will be
                      remembered for this! Vaya con dios!

(JAVEED *revs the angle grinder and moves toward* MIGUEL's *chest*)

MIGUEL   Wait!

JAVEED   What is it? Are you having second
                      thoughts?

MIGUEL   No! I'm wide awake!

JAVEED   Good point. Gas!

KRISTINE   Oh, right, sorry.

(KRISTINE *holds the mask to* MIGUEL's *face and turns the gas on.*
MIGUEL *gets a dreamy look on his face, then conks out*)

JAVEED   Here we go!

Dr. Brewer had smiled at the mention of the Medicus logo on the
heart-lung machine, and had tapped his feet as we sang the song. He
had dabbed tears from his eyes when Kristine prayed over Miguel and
now he was on the edge of his seat.

"Then, as Javeed revs the angle grinder and moves toward Miguel's
chest," I said, "The door to the apartment is suddenly kicked in! We

can see someone is flailing behind the sheets and a voice, off stage, yells, 'Police! You're all under arrest!'"

I clapped my hands loudly and said, "Black out! End of scene."

***

Dr. Brewer sat there, staring at me in pie-eyed wonder. He looked over to Miguel, then back at me. "No, don't stop," he said. "I have to know what happens next!"

"Well," I said, improvising. "We're thrown in jail to await our trial on charges of attempted murder!" I really had no idea what came next since this was as far as I had written the story, but I thought a scene set in jail sounded good and ripe with possibilities. "And then, of course, the trial itself."

"How does it end? You have to tell me."

"Well," I said, "Not to be cagey about it but the fact is there will be no end, or middle, or beginning for that matter unless we have investors first."

"Yes, of course," Dr. Brewer said. "Oh, by the way, I thought the product placement on the bypass machine was a nice touch. Maybe you could do it again when Miguel says he's high as a mountain goat, you know? Mention one of our cannabis products?"

"Absolutely," I said. "Excellent suggestion."

Yes, if you want to make a thing of it, I was willing to go so low as to allow product placement on stage, sue me.

Dr. Brewer looked at Miguel and said, "You look a bit... worn out. Are you feeling OK?"

I explained about how the brain tumor caused periodic seizures and that Miguel had suffered one this morning.

"Have you tried CBD?" Dr. Brewer went to one of several cabinets behind his desk and opened it. The shelves were stocked with Medicus Group cannabis products.

"No," Miguel said. "But I'm willing to try…"

"I recommend the pharmaceutical grade over the so-called artisanal stuff," Dr. Brewer said. "It provides about four times the level of CBD and studies have shown it's much more effective in reducing…"

Dr. Brewer was dropping products into a gift bag and seemed to have forgotten he was in the middle of a sentence so I said, "Effective in reducing…"

"Hmm? Oh, yes, in reducing the frequency and intensity of seizures," Dr. Brewer said. "Now I don't know if they've been tested on the sort of seizures you experience, but…" Again he drifted off.

"But what's the harm?" I said.

"Exactly!" Dr. Brewer looked at me and said, "How about you?"

"No, my health is fine, thanks, but…" I craned my neck for a look into the cabinet.

"How about some of our recreational products then? A lot of creative types swear by these." Dr. Brewer filled a second gift bag with edibles, concentrates, and pre-rolled joints.

"Miguel, I've put some literature in your bag, so be sure to share that with your doctor," Dr. Brewer said. "The literature, not the products."

Miguel took the bag. "Thanks, I'll let you know how it goes."

"Wonderful," Dr. Brewer said. "Now, back to business. One of the reasons I asked to meet with you is that I think Miguel's story is fascinating. As you may know, I have a medical background." He went to another cabinet in his office, this one larger than the first. "The other reason is that I have…" Dr. Brewer fumbled for a key to unlock the cabinet and again seemed to forget he had been speaking.

I prompted him with, "The other reason is…"

"Hmm? Oh, yes."

Dr. Brewer unlocked the cabinet, opened it, and gestured at the contents as though it was trouble incarnate. In fact it was cold, hard cash. Great sheaves and stacks of it, so much I could smell it from across the room.

"The other reason is that owing to Federal banking laws, I'm stuck with piles of cash I can't put in the bank. So while I know you're looking for an investor, the question I have is: Would cash be acceptable?"

"To theatre people? Oh good lord yes," I said.

***

"That's good to hear," Dr. Brewer said. "I've got so much of this piling up around here it's a damn fire hazard."

"Of course it's none of my business," I said, "but out of curiosity… how much of a problem are we talking about?"

"It's something like three hundred thousand a month in cash stacking up around here and it's just a mess," Dr. Brewer said. "A hot chocolate mess and I just wish I could get it all cleaned up, you know? It's crazy."

"I can't imagine the trouble, having all that around," I said. "But I'm sure we'll be able to find a nice *tidy* way to make this work for everybody."

I'm no criminal mastermind, but it was perfectly clear what we were talking about and I didn't have the slightest problem with it. Being a producer isn't for Boy Scouts, after all. Dr. Brewer and I went back and forth for a few minutes making vague references to common accounting practices, keeping in mind at all times not to say anything you wouldn't want coming up at a deposition. Then I told a clever joke about the usefulness of shell companies and Dr. Brewer regaled us with an amusing anecdote about a friend who had successfully pulled some wool during an audit. That sort of thing.

In the end it was perfectly clear that we understood we were going to engage in behavior that could be mischaracterized as money laundering, but only by a soulless and overzealous examiner who had it in for patrons of the arts.

When Dr. Brewer finally asked for a ballpark figure, I gave him one large enough to test his mettle and he didn't so much as blink. I told him I would work up a formal budget for the project and would be in touch.

Miguel was exhausted, so I dropped him at his place before getting to work on a couple of press releases to help keep our project in the public eye. The first went out to the Associated Press and the reporters from the *L.A. Times* and *Sacramento Bee*, who had done stories on Miguel.

The release explained how the Superior Court had, without explanation, callously rejected Miguel's altruistic offer to sacrifice himself for the good of eight other citizens. It went on to say that Miguel had taken this terrible news in characteristic stride and had found it in his heart to forgive the State's attorney and the judge for their parts in the deaths of those who, thanks to their efforts, wouldn't benefit from his organs.

The next release went out to *Variety*, *Hollywood Reporter*, and an assortment of online entertainment news outlets. I sent it out under a phony by-line, as if written by an aspiring entertainment reporter hoping for employment by the big boys.

"According to sources who weren't authorized to speak publicly on the matter, Broadway producer Leonard Stratten is in talks with the August Playhouse regarding the so-called 'Padilla project' (#organguy!). Word is TV phenom Rebecca Vaughn is on board in a starring role and that Stratten was recently seen at a posh Hollywood eatery discussing financing with an unnamed entrepreneur looking to make inroads in the business."

When I finished, I had to pause to marvel at my preposterous good fortune. While I had believed in the value of Miguel's story from the very beginning, I had expected more of an uphill battle to get even a single element working in my favor. In fact I had never expected the whole thing to come together at all. I had serious doubts anyone else would share my vision or see the wisdom in being involved in staging a story such as Miguel's in the manner I was suggesting.

I mean, the man wants the State to carve him into pieces and I want to have people on stage singing about it!

Truth be told, and I hesitate to do so lest you get the wrong impression, my original plan was to swoop in while the story was hot, get the rights to it, then coax some theatre-crazy investor into parting with some dough before everyone cooled on the idea leaving me free to abscond with the remaining cash. Not exactly the crime of the century but it had seemed like a good idea at the time, and it had worked before so, why not?

But to my eternal surprise, piece after piece kept falling into place. Every time I tried to write a more ridiculous song or ramp up the play's absurdity, people seemed even more drawn to it than before. If that weren't bad enough, I had grown terribly fond of Miguel and his friends, which made walking away difficult. And then, to cap things off, I had stumbled into the arms of a morally flexible gentleman who not only loved the story but is literally running out of space to store all of his cash and needs my help.

Now I was trapped, in a manner of speaking. I would actually have to produce the damn thing instead of stealing away in the night with a modest cash infusion. Don't misunderstand, I was looking forward to the task and I thought the script was terrific, but frankly it was hard to believe this was happening.

Of course I still needed an ending for the story, and I wanted to write a new song, but all things considered, things were coming up roses.

Funny how things work out.

15

Ever since Rebecca Vaughn posted about our project, camps had formed and people who had never given a moment's thought about either subject had suddenly staked out unassailable positions on organ donation and physician-assisted death.

You may recall earlier I said there was really no one philosophically opposed to organ donation. But apparently I spoke too soon. On the Internet all claims will be disputed. If you dare post that <<Kittens are cute!>> you are quickly and viciously attacked for ignoring the horrors of feline leukemia and heartworm.

So it was with this.

It was a crackpot contingency to be sure, but, there being no shortage of crackpots out there, anyone who posted something positive about organ donation was immediately confronted by someone from the tin-hat brigade.

<<First of all, you're an idiot! Anybody who has done the research LIKE I HAVE knows the GLOBALISTS are implanting chips into the transplanted organs so they can track and control you! Wake up! If you don't SUBMIT and do what they want, the organ gets rejected! Duh! Donating PERPETUATES the GLOBALIST agenda! Only SUCKERS donate! #organguydie!>>

A post such as this would be followed by dozens of foaming-at-the-mouth comments and eventually hijacked by someone selling a product they claimed would disable the chips implanted by the globalist organ cabal.

And while there was a bakery truck full of those fruitcakes out there, it was the activists opposed to patient autonomy for end-of-life decisions that seized Ethan Cheney's attention. He'd been reading all about what was going on. He was stunned when he discovered that liberal euthanasia squads, at the direction of Deep State operatives, were methodically scouring the state of Oregon, rounding up the handicapped and what they called "hoards of defectives," forcing them to sign postdated(!) documents requesting lethal drugs and then being put down at the request of family members tired of caring for them.

<<It happened to a friend's second cousin!>>

When Ethan Chaney read about this he felt the air leave his lungs.

"Defectives?" Ethan followed that thread and learned that they're trying to kill anyone who isn't a "productive member of society." They're trying to weed out anybody leeching on the system. It was about the money, just like that guy said. Follow the threads!

Ethan Chaney was on disability. He had to be. Wasn't his fault. He couldn't work with his PTSD and his blast-induced traumatic brain injury. So he got a monthly government check. My god, Ethan thought, that's how they'll track me down. And then what?

Something had to be done, Ethan Chaney thought. And he was going to be the one to do it. Someone had to stop the #cultureofdeath!

***

After sampling some of Dr. Brewer's goods I had intended to start working on the script again, searching for the theme of my next song, but I couldn't tear my eyes from the television.

I had stumbled across an animated program starring an optimistic sponge, a red crab, and a squirrel that somehow lived underwater amidst an odd cast of characters. The plot was vexing and character motivations were unclear, but I found myself mesmerized for the longest time.

Fortunately the chime of an incoming text brought me back from the floor of the Pacific Ocean. Kristine had remembered the angle on the property argument that had escaped her after our drunken night at ICU. We were all summoned to Miguel's that night for the reveal.

On my way to Miguel's I stopped at Taco Bistro to pick up a Family Platter, an assortment of their famous street tacos, along with chips and three salsas. Miguel had cold beer waiting for us and he seemed quite cheerful which was a relief to see.

He said he had fully recovered from the exhaustion caused by his seizure and that he had taken some of the CBD that Dr. Brewer had given him. "I don't know if it's a placebo effect or legit," he said, "but I feel calmer and less under attack by my body, if that makes sense."

Reflecting on my time spent with the optimistic sponge and his friends, I said, "I can report without hesitation that his THC products are completely legitimate." No one asked for details, so I offered none.

After parceling out the chips and tacos, we got down to business with Kristine explaining her thinking on a new lawsuit.

"It was something Javeed said after Miguel got that text offering thirty thousand for a kidney," Kristine said. "You were talking about tissue banks and said that bodies and parts are bought, sold, and leased, over and over again."

"Yeah, so?"

"So, it's property!"

"What are you talking about?"

"I'm talking about chattel!"

I wasn't sure I understood, so I said, "What do cows have to do with this?"

"I said chattel," Kristine said. "Not cattle."

"Chattel?"

"Chattel is property," Kristine said. "And when you have property, you have property rights. Rights that are exigible against the world!" She took an enthusiastic bite of her taco.

"So cattle can be chattel?" Javeed said.

"Yes!" Kristine said. "But the more important question is, what about your organs?" She pushed away from the table and started pacing the room. "I mean, think about it. They have all the characteristics of property, don't they? You can touch them, feel them, transfer them to others, exclude others from them. And if that's the case, the state is interfering with your property rights and we will not stand for it!"

"So we're going to sue the bastards again?"

"Exactly!" Kristine went to her purse, pulled out her phone, and said, "Alexa, find characteristics of property." She selected the top result from the search and read aloud, "Personal property includes items intended for personal use." She pointed at Miguel. "Are you using that pancreas?"

"Yeah, as far as I know," he said.

"There you go, that's personal use." She continued reading. "Anything that yields utility or satisfaction to a person. How are your lungs?"

Miguel took a deep breath, and said, "Both utilitarian and satisfying."

"Check," Kristine said. "And were they gained in a socially fair manner?"

"I didn't steal them if that's what you're implying," Miguel said.

"And are you the first person to secure that liver and make use of it?"

"Let's hope so."

"That satisfies the Rule of Capture," Kristine said. "No, wait, that's for natural resources like oil." She waved her hands. "Never mind, doesn't matter, everything about your organs meets the definition of personal property and in matters of personal property, there are inherent rights to protect the property owner."

Javeed said, "What does exigible mean?"

"Enforceable! No one has a right to interfere with your property. And you have the right to do with your property as you wish, provided you don't interfere with the rights of others."

Kristine held a hand out toward Miguel and moved it in a circular motion as if gesturing at his entirety. "Miguel, who does all of that belong to?"

"What, me?"

"Not 'you.' 'You' are more of an abstract thing," Kristine said. "A collection of experiences and memories, things you can't touch or feel or transfer to a third party. I'm talking about your physical self, your body, your... parts. Who do they belong to?

"Well, they're mine, right?"

Kristine cocked her head and said, "Who else could they belong to? No one!"

Miguel was intrigued. "And you can treat your parts like property?"

"Well, you can and you can't," Kristine said. "See, that's where this gets interesting."

"It's true," Javeed said. "You can sell your blood, your plasma, your eggs, your sperm, your... shit."

Miguel turned to Javeed. "What's wrong?"

"What? No, I'm just saying you can sell your shit now. Used to be you couldn't give it away, but fecal microbiota transplants are big business these days," Javeed said. "Stool banks are actually a thing."

I was tempted to make a joke about ATM deposits, but refrained.

"I don't know." Miguel seemed skeptical. "The whole property thing seems like a stretch."

"Of course it is!" Kristine said. "The whole case is a stretch! I wouldn't bother with it if it wasn't a stretch! That's how things change! That's how new law is made, not to mention new law partners."

"So do you have a plan?"

"I did some research," Kristine said. "There are a few cases we might be able to piggyback on. One of them is Moore v. Regents, the result of which was the Court of Appeals ruling that blood and tissue samples *were* personal property."

If I might interrupt, purely in the interest of saving time... Kristine and Javeed then went off on a windy digression related to a woman by the name of Henrietta Lacks and the so-called immortal HeLac cell line. An interesting story, no doubt and not unrelated to the case at hand, but I want to move things forward more quickly than I could possibly recap their discussion. Still, if you're interested, the story has been told in a play, a book, and a film starring Oprah Winfrey.

"And there was Flynn v. Holder," Kristine said. "A case involving bone marrow that moved things forward a bit."

"What happened?"

"A lawyer happened, that's what!" Kristine said. "A lawyer showed up and then, instead of being forced to donate bone marrow, volunteers got paid, like three thousand dollars a visit."

"But it couldn't be cash," Javeed said. "Payment had to be like a health care card or something."

"Yeah, something about the cash makes them squirm," Kristine said. "But the point is, the court said you could sell another part of your body."

"But I'm not trying to sell my organs," Miguel said. "I'm trying to donate them."

"Which is only something you can do with property," Kristine said. "And one thing we will not stand for in this country, is anyone interfering with our property!"

Once again, I was struck as if by lightning and, pounding my fists onto the table top, I shouted, "That's it!"

Javeed was so shocked by my outburst that he dropped his taco and said, "You have *got* to stop doing that!" He put the filling back into the tortilla. "And what are you talking about?"

"It's property!" I said.

They looked at me strangely. "Yes, Leonard, that's what we've been saying for the last ten minutes."

"No, no, not the legal business," I said with a dismissive wave of my hand. "I'm talking about the song. It's about property! Who does it belong to? Is it for sale? This is fantastic! It's the theme I've been searching for. It's about merchandise!"

As sometimes happens in moments of creative fervor I held my hands in front of myself and wiggled my fingers. I don't know why I do this but it seems to be associated with artistic outbursts and somehow helps me connect with my muse. "I'm thinking something uptempo, certainly, possibly Ragtime or Dixieland jazz style. I can hear a sprightly strummed banjo, setting the rhythm. Something along the lines of 'Bourbon Street Parade,' perhaps, or…"

As I mused aloud about the song, trying to think of what might rhyme with "commodity," Javeed slipped into the kitchen without my seeing him. He returned a moment later, behind my back, holding two saucepan lids as if they were a pair of cheap tin crash cymbals.

"Oh," I said. "How about 'oddity'?"

Javeed crashed the two lids together and I nearly jumped out of my skin.

"See?" he smirked.

***

"I could have had a heart attack!"

Javeed seemed pleased with himself and allowed Kristine to snatch the pot lids from his hands as he said, "Let's call it even then."

My phone's chime offered an acceptable pretext to abandon the spat with Javeed. I read the message with delight. "It's from Rebecca Vaughn," I announced. "She says Ace Studios is, and I quote, super excited about the project and they want us to come in for a pitch."

Miguel was thrilled. "Text her back," he said. "Tell her you're writing a new song and ask if she'll pitch with us and sing it."

As I fired off my reply to Rebecca, Kristine returned to her thoughts on Flynn v. Holder, explaining how the Court of Appeals found that the government could reasonably conclude it was morally wrong to sell bone marrow.

"Wait a second," Miguel said. "If it's legal to sell your blood and—"

"The law is a world filled with contradictions," Kristine said. "The court said that allowing the sale of marrow would turn human beings into commodities which was unacceptable."

Javeed laughed at this. "I assume they're unaware of every sports league in America then…"

"Out of curiosity," Miguel said. "What was the rationale for making it illegal to compensate donors in the first place?"

"Funny you should ask," Kristine said. "Because at first they didn't. The guy who chaired the drafting committee said 'compensation should be left to the decency of human beings.' So they sidestepped the question which had also raised concern that the poor would be coerced by financial pressure into selling their organs."

I had already started writing the new song so was listening with only one ear, but that was all it took. I said, "Excuse me, but unless I'm missing something, that would imply it would be acceptable for the wealthy to sell their organs if they wanted, since it wouldn't be due to financial pressure. Do I have that right?"

"Roughly, yes."

"Good," I said. "And now that I have your attention, can anyone think of a word that rhymes with 'product'?" There followed a moment of silence before I said, "Neither can I."

"So when did it become illegal?"

"About twenty-five years later," Kristine said. "After a guy named Jerry Macombs testified to Congress that he intended to start the International Kidney Exchange. The business model, he said, was to buy kidneys from the poor around the world for whatever price would induce them to sell their organs."

"Seriously? Who was this guy?"

"Dr. Jerry Macombs," Kristine said. "Well, Mr. Macombs, after his license was revoked for Medicare fraud. Congress then updated

UAGA with NOTA in 1984 which put the kibosh on compensating donors."

"Damn," I said. "Nothing rhymes with Macombs either."

"This is all very interesting," Miguel said. "But I don't see how it helps since I'm not trying to sell my organs." He paused. "Unless of course the state makes that the only way I can donate them."

"I'm not sure either," Kristine said. "Flynn failed with Due Process and Equal Protection, just like we did with the conflicting laws. So I'm hoping to find an argument about the state interfering with your personal property for no good reason."

Elbows on the table, Javeed steepled his fingers and said, "So NOTA specifically says blood and sperm and bone marrow and other stuff are property but that organs aren't?"

"Right."

"So we need a way to find a way to prove that they are," Javeed said.

"I'm listening."

"Property is something you can steal, right?"

"Yeah," Kristine said, "that's one of the characteristics."

"I have an idea."

***

The plan was simple yet daring. It had to be; we had only six hours to put it together. With the help of a sympathizer inside St. Luke's, we learned of an organ harvest scheduled at their facility for later that night.

The donor was a man named Jimmy Thrush. Not being a Nine-to-Five type, Jimmy cooked some meth and wrote bad checks to keep the wolves from the door. He was an independent-minded sort who wore a red ball cap, enjoyed fast food, beer, and tinkering in his garage.

That afternoon, Jimmy had planned to weld a set of super loud pipes onto his Harley. Neighbor-haters, he called them. That's just the kind of guy he was.

Jimmy had learned flux-core and shielded-metal arc welding before he was kicked out of trade school for stealing equipment. But he wouldn't have stayed long anyway since he couldn't tolerate people telling him how to do things like mixing dangerous gasses.

Jimmy preferred thinking outside the box. And today was no exception. Today he was going to try his latest experimental welding kit. He had put a mixture of acetylene and oxygen, the standard ingredients used in oxy-fuel welding, into a liquid propane gas bottle.

Now, your typical know-it-all will keep these components in separate tanks because, when combined, they burn hot enough to cut metal, but not Jimmy. He was a tough guy with a libertarian streak. And in another nod to his Don't-Tread-On-Me mentality, Jimmy had fashioned his kit without a flow regulator. Hell yeah. Jimmy was a lifetime subscriber to the notion that government regulations were the problem not the solution.

He was tickled pink by the looks of his jury-rigged device and couldn't wait to give it try. So he attached a torch head straight to the bottle and lit the welding tip.

Lacking a regulator, the flame crept back into the bottle and the inevitable explosion spread his garage, which also contained about ten gallons of paint thinner and gasoline, throughout the neighborhood.

While the explosion relieved Jimmy of both of his hands and did some other damage, it somehow didn't kill him. He was, however, in what the neurologist at St. Luke's would call the deepest irreversible coma she had ever seen. Asked about the odds of Jimmy regaining consciousness, the doctor said her own great, great, great-grandfather had a better chance of coming back to life.

Fortunately for some people on the waiting lists, Jimmy had done one good thing in his life which was to check the organ donor box when he got his class M-1 license, which had expired two years earlier but without invalidating his status as an organ donor.

Unfortunately, Jimmy's liver was shot so it was going into the trash but everything else was in surprisingly good shape. His heart was being airlifted to San Diego, his lungs to Bakersfield, one kidney was headed for San Francisco and the other was destined for Ascendant Medical on the far side of the L.A. Medical Complex.

This would be our target.

Javeed showed us the route the courier would have to take, essentially circling the perimeter of the complex and entering a service road that led to the back of Ascendant Medical where he would be met by someone from the transplant team who would receive the organ and confirm delivery with a simple bar scan.

There were three side streets that fed into the service road which allowed us to set our trap. Kristine was parked on one of them, in a poorly lit area between two distant streetlights. She was waiting there for our call.

The harvest started on time so we moved into position. The courier from Terrific Tissue Transport was driving a blue minivan marked with the T-3 logo. We saw him exit the building carrying a teal-blue special edition Scooby-Doo Mystery Machine seven-quart Igloo cooler. It was a versatile nine-can cooler with the iconic tent-top design, perfect for tailgating or kidney transport.

The courier secured the cooler in the passenger seat and did a U-turn out of the loading zone.

We could only hope he was unarmed.

We kept our distance as we followed and called Kristine when the time was right. She pulled out from the side street, blocking the service road ahead of the courier. She popped the trunk and grabbed her jumper cables, then opened the hood of her car and leaned over the engine to connect the cable clamps to the battery terminals.

The courier, being a courteous type who had a few minutes owing to the generous ischemic time for kidneys, nosed the minivan up to give Kristine a jump. He got out to offer assistance, opening the minivan's hood to access the battery. This also blocked his vision enough that he didn't notice when Miguel pulled up behind him.

We pulled our ski masks over our faces and slipped from the car. Miguel went to the driver's side. He was going to unlock the doors, kill the engine, take the keys and the courier's phone. I went to the passenger side to snatch the cooler.

We opened the doors simultaneously and in a second I had the cooler in hand. Miguel looked around the interior and said, "No keys! He's got the fob with him, and his phone."

This threw our plan into disarray. Killing the engine wouldn't do much good if they guy could start it right back up. And if he had his phone, he could call the cops before we had a chance to get very far.

"What do we do?"

"You drive my car," Miguel said. "I'll take this one and—"

"Hey!" The courier had seen us. "What the hell are you doing?" That's when he pulled his gun. "Put that down, now!" He motioned with the gun.

"Wait!" I froze, one hand in the air. "I can explain!"

"Put it down!" He raised the gun, pointing it directly at me. "Now!"

"This isn't what it looks like!" Miguel said.

The courier's finger moved toward the trigger and he fired a shot, wildly, missing both of us by a mile as he screamed in pain.

Kristine had clamped the jumper cables onto the courier's neck. He dropped the gun, collapsing in a heap, the cables still gripping his flesh. He twitched and jerked like it was a grand mal seizure before coming to a stop a moment later.

Kristine removed the clamps and looked at him.

"Is he OK?" I asked.

Miguel shook his head. "He doesn't look good."

Kristine was gripped with fear. "Oh my god," she said. "I killed him."

"Whoa, Kristine, calm down, he was pointing a gun at me," I said. "You were defending me."

"Oh my god, no! It's worse than that!" Kristine shrieked. "I killed him during the commission of a robbery. That's special circumstances. That's felony murder. I'll be executed!"

Kristine heard the sirens approaching. She wheeled and pointed accusingly at us. "And not just me! You two are accomplices! We're all going to fry!"

16

Ashley Winters, the Head of Production at Ace Studios said, "That's a great scene but how are you going to do it on the stage, I mean the cars and everything?"

"No, no, the stealing-the-kidney scene is just for the film," I said. "In the stage version we all end up in jail for attempted murder after trying to harvest Miguel's organs in his living room."

"Oh," Ashley said. "Got it."

"That's a very funny scene too," Rebecca Vaughn said. "And it has another great song in it." She hopped to her feet and did a little of the old song and dance: "My kidney's failin'... man I'm ailin'... the pain's off the chart!"

Rebecca, Miguel, and I were in Ashley Winter's office on the Ace Studios lot in Culver City, along with one of Ashley's assistants, a young man named Liam.

"So yes," I said. "Obviously, there will be a lot of differences between a film version and what we can do on the stage." I explained about the television screens. "I wish I could think of a way to do that in the film but, so far, that just doesn't work. It's a theatrical thing and it just doesn't translate."

Liam said, "You know a twelve-volt car battery really won't shock you like that," he said. "They have the amperage, but not the volts."

Ashley looked at her assistant. "No one cares, Liam," she said. "It's an accepted film trope. This isn't a fucking documentary."

I smiled. "You wouldn't believe how many times I have to say that to people."

"Rebecca, I think you were born to play the Kristine part,' Ashley said. "The feisty lawyer, smart, capable, and loyal to your dying friend…"

"And willing to commit a crime to prove it," Rebecca said. "I can't tell you how excited I am about this project! It's serious and funny and… the songs! It's just so original!"

"OK," Ashley said. "So what happens next?"

"The police arrive and arrest us," I said.

"Is the courier dead?" Liam asked. "Because a car battery really can't—"

"No, he's fine," I said. "He comes to."

"Forget the damn battery," Ashley said before turning to me with a smile. "Please, don't mind Liam, he's simple and possibly heading back to the mail room. Go on."

"Now, I'm going to give you the stage version of this scene since I've developed it more fully," I said. "The film version will just be a variation on this."

"Of course."

I framed the scene with my hands and said, "Cut to: Our day in court. The judge saying the defendants are charged with conspiracy to commit murder and attempted murder in the first degree. How do you plead?

"Here, my character stands and says, 'Your Honor, if I might? Leonard Stratten for the accused.'

"'You're one of them,' the judge says. 'Do you have any legal training?'

"'Not as such, Your Honor, but I directed an extended run of *Witness for the Prosecution* off-Broadway.'

"'Did you? Wonderful play.'

"'Yes, Your Honor, and in light of that I must say that none of us should even be here. You see, I heard about this poor boy's story and went to secure the dramatic rights for an opera I intend to produce.'

"'Oh,' the judge says, 'I love opera.'

"'Yes, Your Honor, and this one is becoming increasingly tragic. In any event, I made a good faith offer of half a million dollars for the rights—'

"Miguel bolts to his feet at this. 'Objection! He offered a full million!'

"'It's still a million, of course,' I say, waving a comforting hand. 'But a lot of that is on the back end. It's very common.'

"'Objection overruled,' the judge says. 'He's right, they do that sort of thing all the time.'

"'Thank you, Your Honor. So, as I was saying, we were merely engaged in a rehearsal for the big scene when the constables kicked in the door and arrested us.'

"The judge says, 'And you bought an actual heart-lung bypass machine for this rehearsal?'

"'Your Honor, I freely admit the staging and set design and even some of the performances were magnificent, especially in light of the budget and level of talent with which I had to work, but the idea we were seriously engaged in attempted murder is utterly ridiculous.'

"'Well, this whole thing is utterly ridiculous, if you ask me,' the judge says. 'Nonetheless, here we are.'

"'I couldn't agree more, Your Honor,' I say. 'And in keeping with that, I would like to give you a sneak peek at one of the numbers my co-defendants and I worked up for the musical while we were rotting in the slammer.'

"'Musical? I thought you said it was an opera.'

"'Suffice to say there will be some singing, Your Honor.'

"'Well,' the judge says, 'This is highly unusual, but yes, by all means, proceed.'

"Here I motion to the bailiff in the back of the courtroom and say to the judge, 'Your Honor, I would like to introduce Exhibit A.' All eyes turn to look as the bailiff rolls a portable Hammond into the courtroom.

"The judge says, 'A piano?'"

"'An organ, Your Honor. Get it? Organ?'

"'Mr. Stratton,' the judge says, 'This court has given you a great deal of leeway, but another pun such as that and I will find you in contempt!'

"'It won't happen again, Your Honor,' I say. 'Now if it pleases the court, my co-defendants and I will do a number based on the Hughie Cannon standard, "Won't You Come Home Bill Bailey?" Think of it as an ode to the Ninth Circuit's ruling on Flynn v. Holder as regards the question of property.'

"'How exciting,' the judge says.

"At this point I sit at the Hammond and play a couple of bars before Miguel comes in singing:

'Who owns my kidney, honey?

Who owns my spleen?

I like to think they're mine.

I'll trade 'em for some money,

Won't that be keen?

I'll make the big headline.'

"Rebecca takes the next part:

'Remember that the courts are saying, that's not for sale.

That heart's not merchandise they said.

No transplants, it's a shame.

And tell me who's to blame?

We're sorry but some end up dead.'

"I begin to play a kazoo as Miguel and Kristine trade this one-off line by line.

'She needs a transplant, baby.

He needs one too.

But parts are getting hard to find.
Get on the list and maybe,
You won't be through.
But someone will be left behind.'
"Rebecca sings the final chorus.
    'Remember you can sell your blood cells and rent your womb,
But then they start to draw that line.
They'll throw you into jail,
No money man, no bail.
And you'll just have to serve your time...'"

***

My apologies if there was any confusion about what just happened just now. Please allow me to clarify.

A couple of days ago, when we were discussing the legal possibilities of human organs being property, Javeed floated the notion that we steal an organ in order to find out what charges would be proposed by the investigating officer. The idea being that if the officer classified it as theft or robbery it would prove that we were dealing with property since property is the only thing one can steal or rob. This would be evidence Kristine could use in the course of the lawsuit.

Since we weren't interested in finding out what charges might be pressed if the kidney patient died waiting for the organ, Javeed insisted that after stealing the kidney, we would take it immediately to the hospital personnel waiting for it, explaining that the courier's vehicle had broken down and had asked us to deliver the organ.

While we all agreed Javeed's idea was well worth considering, we also agreed there were too many things that could go wrong so we decided against actually doing it. However, I recognized it as an excellent scene to include in the film pitch to Ashley Winters so that's what we did the next day when we were at Ace Studios.

And if you're curious, I gave the organ donor in the scene a simple backstory because it's something I do instinctively when I'm telling tales.

In any event, when we finished singing "The Property Song," Ashley Winters seemed somewhat befuddled, which I took as a bad sign. She shook her head in disbelief and said, "Well, this is a first." She didn't sound pleased about it either.

Miguel, Rebecca, and I looked at one another apprehensively, not sure what to make of the comment. Finally, I said, "In what way?"

Ashley assumed the posture of a corporate media titan and said, "Ace Studios takes a somewhat cautious approach when acquiring material, or maybe thoughtful is a better word." She looked at Liam, who nodded solemnly in agreement. "We like to bring in the various department heads, marketing, finance, and so forth, to get their input before committing ourselves to a project. I'm sure you understand."

"Of course," I said. "You'd like us to come back and pitch to a larger room?"

"No," Ashley smiled. "As I said, this is a first. I'm giving the green light now," she said, breaking into a smile.

Rebecca leaped to her feet with a "Whoop!" She gave Miguel a big hug, then Ashley, then me. Liam, situated, as he was, at the bottom of the totem pole, got a fist bump.

It wasn't an unconditional green light, but the conditions weren't onerous either. Ashley said she liked the idea I had pitched at our first meeting with Rebecca and her agent, Robin Harris, at CIA: Get the play staged, see how it runs. If it's a hit, we make a film, which, if it's a hit, spawns a sequel and a television series. And, of course, a soundtrack album that I would produce.

***

Ever since the Lynn Mitchum interview and the announcement that #organguy! was headed for the stage, Miguel's story had seized the public's and the media's attention.

So when Kristine filed the new lawsuit, the *L.A. Times* moved the story from the Law and Politics section to the front page. The story noted that Miguel was again challenging the State's interference with his right to donate his organs. The reporter recapped the court's decision on the previous suit and went on to speculate on how the new suit might successfully challenge the National Organ Transplant Act and bring about a long-overdue update on the Uniform Anatomical Gift Act.

Asked for a comment, a spokesperson for Southern California Organ Procurement Enterprises did a delicate dance saying that Miguel's case was both tragic and legally fraught and that everyone in the organization wished Miguel the best. He refused to go on record about the organization's reaction to Miguel's request to be harvested to death, but off-the-record noted that it would be a terrible shame if the organs went to the grave instead of to saving lives.

There was a sidebar story that delved into the medical ethics of Miguel's request, citing opposing views from the nation's most well-known medical ethicists, none of whom anyone had ever heard of. I gave up after sampling a dense passage about consequentialist versus intrinsic corruption and the inherent incompatibility between an object and a mode of valuation.

The reporter wrapped the story up by noting that Miguel's case had inflamed passions among members of the organ donation and transplantation community as well as those in favor of, and opposed to, patient autonomy.

Meanwhile, in the Entertainment section of the *Times*, we had a second story courtesy of Ashley Winters who put out a press release announcing that Ace Studios had given the green light to the film version of "The Padilla Project #organguy!" with Rebecca Vaughn in a starring role and co-producer credit (which was news to me). Rebecca was quoted as saying she was extremely excited about the project, given that organ donation was her pet cause and because the script was so unique with its blend of drama, humor, and music.

The moment these stories hit the Internet, Ethan Chaney's phone chimed. He had a news alert set for any mention of Miguel's name or #organguy!

The article about Ace Studio's plan to make a movie about Miguel Padilla grated on Ethan Chaney's nerves because he just knew Hollywood would present this act of depravity as some sort of valiant effort to save innocent lives and would portray Miguel as a hero instead of being just another pawn in the culture of death.

This was a dispiriting turn of events, but the movie was too far in the future to require immediate action or any more of Ethan's attention.

The story about the start of the lawsuit, on the other hand, gave Ethan Chaney an idea. He had to do something to stop Miguel and his supporters from getting what they wanted. And what they wanted was to legitimize the Deep State liberal euthanasia agenda even further.

Ethan Chaney was ready to answer this call-to-arms. It would be self-defense, really, since he knew the euthanasia squads could be kicking in his door any day now.

Ethan needed to gear up and he wasn't going to find what he needed at Walmart. So he dove to the depths of the dark web, where he could acquire the things he needed to fight the battle.

It hadn't been the Army's goal, of course, but all that time they spent teaching Ethan Chaney how to disarm an IED, they were also teaching him how to build one. It's what they call an unintended consequence.

***

People misunderstand what luck is. The dictionary says it's the seemingly chance happening of events. "Seemingly" being the key word for what I have to say here.

Winning the lottery is mostly luck. You do have to make the effort to purchase the ticket so there is some "work" involved, but, let's face it, not much, especially if you let the machine pick the numbers. But beating one-in-fourteen-million odds is about as close to pure luck as you are going to get.

Now, far too many people credit whatever success they have in life to their hard work and savvy, refusing to acknowledge the part luck played in getting where they are. They want all the credit. Human nature, I suppose.

I am not one of those people, at least I try not to be. I understand the role luck plays and it has played the starring role in this particular play, has it not?

I mean, what are the odds that I would get to Miguel first and acquire the rights to his story, that Rebecca Vaughn would join us, that the August Playhouse would be looking for just what we were offering, that a visit to an underground hospital would lead to a meeting with a man who was fascinated by the story and who was drowning in cash, and that a major Hollywood film studio would swoon at our pitch?

The odds are incalculable. One would require tremendous luck for all this to happen, yes?

But, as the saying goes, luck favors the prepared. It seems to reward effort.

I'm reminded of the famous attorney who was asked if luck played any part in success at trial and he said yes, and it usually comes at three in the morning when I'm in the library doing research.

The point being: the more work you put into it, the more luck you have. Which brings us back to that word, "seemingly."

"The seemingly chance happening of events."

Nothing in the series of events I have presented so far happened by pure chance. Everything happened because I worked very hard to create the circumstance where—if I happened to get lucky—I would have success.

These were my thoughts as I strolled down the famous Santa Monica Pier that night, illuminated by the colorful lights of the Ferris wheel and invigorated by the jostle and noise of the crowd.

It almost felt like walking down Broadway.

I continued up to Palisades Park, away from the crowd, where I sauntered past the palm trees, their fronds rustling in a gentle ocean breeze. I was singing softly to myself, "Who owns my kidney, honey? Who owns my spleen? I like to think they're mine…"

I gazed out at the moonlit Pacific thinking that there was nothing left for me to do. I had made the sale. I could finally relax. All that remained was casting and rehearsal. The easy stuff. Oh, we would have to deal with the contracts—the dreaded lawyers—crossing the Ts, dotting the Is, and all that but…

"Excuse me? Aren't you Leonard Stratten, the producer?"

A voice from behind me, one I didn't recognize off the top. I assumed it was someone in the business I had met along the way. I turned and said, "Yes, that's right."

"Well," the man said. "Then I'd like my money back."

"What?"

In the twilight I could see the handgun aimed at me. A semi-automatic from the looks of it.

"And I want it in cash, you thieving bastard."

He stepped out of the shadows enough that I could see.

It was him. "McElheny, old chap!" I said, pointing with my cane. "Just the man I've been looking for!" I didn't know what else to say. "You had me going there for a second. How in the world *are* you?"

"Don't give me that shit," he said. "I want my fifty thousand. Now."

I maintained my composure, hoping for a final bit of luck as I said, "What? No, I thought we'd put that behind us after Mr. Carlton's untimely death. Taken too soon, wouldn't you say?"

"Cut the crap, Stratton. You won't con me twice," McElheny said. "There was no Emmitt Carlton III, no malaria, and no pending million-dollar investment either."

"What?" I said. "I met with Mr. Carlton myself. I showed you the letter from the bank, right? What are you saying?"

"The documents were fake."

"What? Well, if that's the case then I'm the one who was conned, not you," I said. "But let's deal with that later." I stepped a little closer to convey congeniality. "Let me tell you about my new project. It's fantastic! In fact we just got the green light to make a film with Ace Studios. We can just roll your money into this one."

"I almost had you in Mexico," McElheny said. "Then you disappeared again until you went and got your name in the papers."

"Well then, you know I'm on to something good here! A theatre man such as yourself surely recognizes that. And you can have a piece of it to make you whole," I said. "Why don't we go have a drink? I'll tell you all about it."

"I want my money now."

"Well that's a bit unreasonable, isn't it? I mean, who walks around with fifty thousand in cash? Just put the gun away," I said as if it were nothing. "We'll go have a drink and work out the details. What do you say?"

"I say you better come up with the cash."

My only chance was to attract some attention, get some witnesses. I waved at a young couple strolling not too far away. "Hello!" I shouted. "No need to call the police, just a misunderstanding!"

The couple came closer for a better look. This seemed to throw McElheny off a bit, as I'd hoped.

"Cut the bullshit," McElheny said. He motioned with his gun. "Let's go." He tried to steer me into the shadows but I held my ground. I didn't want to die in the dark.

I raised my hands to make it clear to the witnesses there was a crime in progress. I had my cane in one hand, the other was empty. The cane, I thought, would make me look even more the pitiful victim.

When the couple saw my hands go up, one of them pulled his phone and began to record the incident. The other ran off, as if to get help.

"Put your hands down, asshole," McElheny said. "You're drawing attention."

I lowered my voice so that only McElheny could hear me. "What are you waiting for then? I don't have your fifty thousand. You can either take the deal I'm offering or you can piss off."

"Or I can shoot you."

"You don't have what it takes," I said.

The man with the phone said that he had called the cops.

McElheny turned to yell at the man, "Mind your own business or you're next!"

A moment later, I could see the man flinch when he heard the shot.

17

A crowd gathered with their phones to get photos and video of the body sprawled on the grass.

Police arrived within minutes and cordoned off the area. An ambulance came quickly.

The lead officer was examining the weapon when he said, "Where'd you get this?"

"I had it made years ago," I said. "A gunsmith in Philadelphia."

"I've never seen one of these before," the policeman said as he admired the craftsmanship. "Very nice work."

"Yes, it's based on the design of a popular cane gun made in France in the late nineteenth century, though this is thoroughly modern… and legal, I should add."

"What is it, a .22?"

"No, it's a 9mm," I said. "It's breech loaded, you just unscrew the cane here to get to the chamber." I pointed at the part in question. "There's a steel ferrule at the bottom with a cork capping the end so the barrel stays clean."

"Just one shot?"

"Yes, it helps to be close," I said, glancing toward the paramedics. "Am I in some sort of trouble?"

"No." The officer said the witness's video showed it was clearly self-defense, so I wasn't facing any charges. He said, "Did you know the man?"

"Never seen him before," I replied. "Said his name was Emmitt Carlton III."

A patrolman handed McElheny's wallet to the officer.

"Did he try to rob you?"

"Yes, he said he wanted money."

"Weird that he would introduce himself before trying to rob you."

"Yes, well, I tried to engage him in conversation, you know? Trying to talk him down, I suppose. He seemed like he might be high on something and I thought... well, it doesn't really matter what I thought, other than maybe if I were friendly to him..." I shrugged like I had no answers.

The officer held up a driver's license he had plucked from the wallet. "Looks like he lied about his name," the officer said. "ID says it's McElheny, not Carlton."

"How very odd," I said. "I hesitate to ask but, is he... dead?"

"No, but the EMTs don't like his chances."

"Oh, that's bad luck," I said. "Bad luck indeed."

And then, as the ambulance pulled away, I wondered if McElheny had signed his organ donor card.

***

I'm no killer, of course, but I am a survivor. As for McElheny, who knows? Did he have what it takes? Would he have shot me? It didn't seem prudent to find out. I offered him a fair deal to get his money back, after all, but, despite my generous offer, he still seemed intent on doing me harm, so... off he went in the ambulance.

I was torn over the question of whether or not I should go to the press about it. My thinking was that if I went to them with the story, I had some chance of controlling the narrative. It seemed all but certain that the story would break one way or the other. After all, a dashing twenty-first-century man in a stylish suit shooting his assailant with a gun concealed in his nineteenth-century walking cane is a terrific story.

And it seemed possible the story could greatly enhance my reputation in the business. Not only is he handsome and stylish, they would say, but dangerous too. I certainly wouldn't cross him. Even the biggest sharks in town would offer genuine respect.

On the other hand, if some overenthusiastic muckraker decided to dig a bit deeper and look into the background of the man who got shot, he or she might discover McElheny and I had a history. This information would no doubt find its way back to the Santa Monica Police and put me in the position of having to explain why I told them I didn't know the man. And when the cops find out you've lied to them once, everything else you've said gets put under the microscope and who needs that?

But maybe even that would be worth it. I could always walk it back by saying it had been so long since I'd seen McElheny and our history was so scant that I didn't recognize the man. That might fly.

It seemed obvious that the story of a man shooting a stranger who had tried to rob him played well with the public. Pure self-defense, they'd say. Bully for him standing his ground. But the story of a man shooting someone he owed money to, even if it was at gunpoint, well, that water was considerably murkier. But maybe in a good way. Word would spread that I was more dangerous than anyone thought. Don't try anything shady with that guy, they'd say.

But if someone asked the right questions and got pointed in the right direction, the phony bank documents might surface and that might encourage someone to pursue a charge of fraud. And that might be enough to kill the current project. So, in the end, I decided to keep my mouth shut, not even telling my friends about the event. If the story came out anyway, I would just have to deal with it.

***

The night before the trial was set to begin, Kristine gathered us as a sort of focus group to test drive her possible opening statements.

Needless to say, beverages were served.

Kristine took a sip of her tangerita before saying, "Ladies and gentlemen of the jury… Assuming their game plan is the same as the last time we did this, the State will try to convince you that what we want to do is open an unregulated retail organ outlet on every street corner, opposite Starbucks. They want you to imagine a horde of grimy vendors buying and selling entrails at bloody roadside stalls thick with flies while an impoverished family of four slinks away in the background with nothing more than pocket change and stitches in their soon-to-be-infected flanks."

Javeed cast a doubtful glance in my direction.

Kristine pointed at Miguel as she continued, "They want you to believe that if you help Mr. Padilla donate his organs in the unorthodox way he is asking, if you do that, the next thing you know, perfectly healthy Americans will be clamoring to be harvested to death. And they say this is going to happen in a country where almost half the population refuses to even register as a donor! It beggars belief."

She paused here and said, "So? What do you think?"

"It's very… colorful," Miguel said.

"Extremely," Javeed agreed. "Some vivid imagery, for sure. Really grabs your attention."

"Yeah," Kristine said, "but in a good way?"

"Well, that's hard to say," Javeed replied. "As much as I liked it, I wonder if you may be putting in the jury's head the image you're accusing the State of wanting them to have."

"Sort of doing their job for them," Miguel said.

"Oh, OK." Kristine turned to me for my thoughts.

"I think it's wonderful," I said.

"Really?"

"Yes, but I think it's probably better for the play than it is for the courtroom," I said. "It seems a bit… much."

Kristine appeared somewhat wounded by our comments and took another sip on her drink. Then she stated laughing. "You guys are such dupes! Stitches in their soon-to-be-infected flanks? You really think I would use that for an opening statement?"

"Well…"

"That's obviously my closing argument!"

"What?"

"I'm kidding!" Kristine said. "I wrote that for fun. But if you can use it in the play, you're welcome to it."

"Well done," I said. "Now, seriously. What've you got?"

Not surprisingly, Kristine had a raft of excellent ideas. The trick, we decided, was finding our theme, then selecting the best of her ideas to tell the story, and then to assemble the facts in a persuasive sequence. Kristine was a skillful writer and gifted when it came to recognizing a good note versus a bad one.

The four of us sat at the table for hours, laughing and talking and taking Kristine's direction as we wrote, rewrote, edited and polished until we were all satisfied and, once again, a bit drunk. It was a night I will always remember.

***

If I might do some expectation management… I wanted to let you know what you have in store as the trial unfolds. As always, I will filter out the extraneous, the superfluous, and the unnecessary for your convenience, focusing instead on the compelling, the interesting, and the indispensable.

Kristine and Miguel (spoiler alert: he gets to be co-counsel) will guide you and the jury through their arguments about "The body as property," "The principals of Gift Law", and the vital role "Scarcity" plays in the establishment of property rights.

I promise you it's more entertaining than it sounds. So, with that in mind, here's what happened…

Much to my dismay, the new trial was to be held in the same place as the last one, in one of the converted double-wide mobile homes in a satellite parking lot for the California Superior Court in Chatsworth. There were a dozen of these temporary structures spread out over two acres of asphalt. Ours was somewhere in the middle.

On the far edge of the lot I could see people carrying protest signs. As they got closer I could see one: "I HEART Miguel!" And another: "Donate Now!" A third said "TAPAS!", which I assumed was an advertisement for a nearby food truck.

The makeshift courtroom was cramped. The gallery was necessarily small. After making room for the judge's riser, the witness stand, the attorneys' tables, and the jury box there was only room for five narrow rows of public seating. There were a couple of print reporters and several curious members of the public.

Team Miguel was up front: Javeed, Rebecca Vaughn, and I sitting directly behind the plaintiff's table. To my surprise I had passed through Security without a problem and carried my weapon into the courtroom.

After the usual delays, we got down to business.

The jury, finally empaneled and sworn in, listened as Kristine delivered the opening statement we had crafted the night before. She began with some improvisation, mocking the State, suggesting their motives were impure in removing from the jury everyone who had had an organ transplant or had a friend or relative who had.

"But," Kristine said. "They couldn't get rid of everybody who *might* one day need one. Like each of you or your spouse, or your children. So as you listen to the testimony ask yourself how you would feel about the State's position if you or someone you loved *did* need an organ."

Kristine then gave the jury a recap of the first lawsuit, characterizing the decision as one borne of cowardice with the court too timid to venture into the murky wake of Bi-Metallic Investment Company v. State Board of Equalization.

"Ladies and gentlemen, we are here today for one simple reason," Kristine said. "My client, Miguel Padilla, wants to exercise his rights.

And the State of California wants to prevent him from doing so, and not for the first time. You see, the State guaranteed my client – and all of you, for that matter – the right to donate organs without interference. The State also guaranteed my client the right to physician-assisted death in light of his terminal diagnosis."

Kristine leveled an accusing finger at the State's attorney. "But now the State is saying, well, you…" She turned to point at Miguel "… Mr. Padilla, you don't get to exercise your rights like the rest of us because, well, because your case gives us the willies."

Kristine acknowledged that what Miguel was asking for could be construed as disturbing or even grotesque and that the case wasn't one for the squeamish. "But," she said, "my client doesn't think that justifies letting eight people die who don't have to. So we are here to ask for your help in saving their lives."

I caught some movement out of the corner of my eye and glanced over in time to see a brief parade of signs pass by outside the window. "I'm With Miguel!" followed by "My Body, My Property!" and, again, "TAPAS!" This triggered in me the sudden urge for some patatas bravas so I decided I would try to find that food truck at lunch to see if that was on the menu.

Meanwhile, Kristine wrapped up her statement by saying, "I intend to show that my client, Miguel Padilla, has a property interest in the constituent parts of his body and that the State is interfering unnecessarily with his property rights."

The judge peered over the top of her glasses and said, "Your argument will be about people… as property?"

"Yes, Your Honor."

The judge looked to the jury, four of whom were African American, all of whom had rather incredulous expressions on their faces. "You may recall," the judge said, "the last time this country allowed humans to be treated as property it didn't work out very well for a certain segment of the population."

The Black jury members nodded solemnly.

Kristine looked at the jury and said, "Oh, that! Yes. I forgot. Well, not 'forgot' but I hadn't even considered…" She waved her hands frantically. "So, no, that's absolutely not what we are advocating, Your Honor, ladies and gentlemen. We're not arguing that one person should have a property interest in *another* person. We are saying an individual should have a property interest in him or herself and their own parts, as Henrietta Lacks should have had, and as such we should all be free from interference with these property rights."

The jury members seemed satisfied with this explanation and the judge said, "Yes, that would be… decidedly different. You may proceed."

At this point, the State's attorney, a doughy fellow by the name of Ken Stern rose sluggishly to say, "Your Honor, the State is concerned that if donors are allowed to be compensated, the wealthy or the medical industry itself might attempt to coerce the poor into selling their organs."

Kristine said, "And you think the best alternative is to allow organ-procurement specialists to do the coercion instead?"

"I wouldn't characterize what procurement specialists do as coercion," Ken said. "It's more like… persuasion," he said without conviction. "In any case, the State's position is that the idea of property rights in human tissue raises grave concerns that counsel is angling to create a market for organs that would do nothing except exploit the poor."

Kristine said, "Exploit the poor? Everything exploits the poor! You think rich people mine coal and diamonds? No! Rich people get poor people to do that and take all the money. You think payday lenders and regressive taxes don't exploit the poor? Where's your grave concern for the poor then?"

Mr. Stern, having no good answer, sat down glumly just as Miguel stood and said, "We're not trying to establish a market, Your Honor. I don't want to sell my organs. I want to donate them, as is my lawfully guaranteed right."

"All the sudden you're representing yourself?" the judge said.

"Well, they're my parts, Your Honor," Miguel said. "Plus, I aced Civil Procedure. So, if it pleases the court, I'd like to be co-counsel."

"Fine, Mr. Padilla," the judge said. "You may proceed."

"Thank you, Your Honor," Miguel said. "Now, what is personal property according to the law? It has to be a physical thing, tangible, moveable, and transferrable."

Kristine continued, "It is something you can give as a gift and something you can sell and deliver to others."

Mr. Stern rose sluggishly to say, "Objection. Separability, Your Honor. Personal property must be physically separate to the rights holder." He sounded like a man just going through the motions, and reluctantly at that.

Kristine called to the stand Dr. Mark Simmons, renowned cardiologist and transplant surgeon. She asked him if human organs could be separated from a body and transferred to another.

"Yes, of course," Dr. Simmons said. "It's done routinely."

"Objection overruled."

"Now, as long as I have you here, Dr. Simmons, let me ask you a few more questions. Let's say I need a heart transplant," Kristine said. "I reach the top of the list and a donor heart becomes available. Walk me through what happens."

Dr. Simmons said, "The local organ-procurement organization, the O.P.O., acquires the heart from the donor's family and arranges for its transport to the transplant hospital."

"The O.P.O. acquires it for how much, on average?"

"It's always for nothing," Dr. Simmons said. "The donor's family is prohibited from receiving any compensation."

"In accordance with the Uniform Anatomical Gift Act..."

"Yes."

"Thank you, Dr. Simmons," Kristine said. "I don't have any further questions at the moment, but I may be calling you back to the stand later."

Ken Stern, who looked like he would rather be anywhere on earth other than sitting here trying to justify the State's position in this case, said he had no questions for the witness. He then asked for, and was granted, a brief recess which he spent sitting despondently in a bathroom stall despairing about his choice of career.

***

As always, I was making notes as the trial unfolded. The final scene had yet to be written and the question in my mind was whether it would take place in this courtroom or somewhere else. Should it end with the jury's decision? Or, depending on how the jury found, should it end with Miguel being wheeled into the operating room of an accredited hospital or into the underground facility? Or would it be at Miguel's funeral? Each had dramatic possibilities. At this point, I could only wait to see what hand Fate dealt us.

When we returned from the recess, Kristine called to the stand a woman by the name of Terry Putnam, a former associate to the General Counsel for UNOS.

Kristine pulled a small box from her purse. It was wrapped in colorful paper and tied with a red ribbon and bow. She approached the witness, offering the box. "Good afternoon, Ms. Putnam." Kristine handed her the box.

"What's this?" Ms. Putnam asked.

"It's a gift," Kristine said. "Open it."

The jury seemed intrigued by the gambit.

Ms. Putnam opened the box. Inside was a shiny silver paperweight in the shape of a heart. "How nice," she said. "Thank you."

"You're welcome," Kristine said. "Now, Ms. Putnam, what can you tell us about the legal framework governing organ distribution in the United States?"

"Well, as I'm sure you know, the primary law is the Uniform Anatomical Gift Act, which established Gift Law as the central legal principal guiding the U.S. opt-in system of organ donation," Ms. Putnam said. "UAGA was built on the principles of Gift Law and designed to support the system of transplantation."

"And how is that going? The opt-in system?"

"Well, it's going better than one might hope but not as well as one might wish," Ms. Putnam said with a smile.

"Can you tell us what percentage of people who die will do so in a way that allows for organ donation to be a possibility? I would guess, what, sixty or seventy percent?"

"No, unfortunately it's only about two percent."

"Two percent?" Kristine turned to the jury with a shocked expression. "No wonder so many people die waiting. What is it, like twenty people a day?"

"Yes," Ms. Putnam said. "It's less than ideal, but those are the numbers."

"Are those the numbers worldwide, more or less?"

"More or less."

"Can you think of any country in the world where the numbers are significantly better?"

"Yes," Ms. Putnam said. "Iran."

"Iran? Interesting. And do you know why their numbers are so much better?"

"Yes, it's because they have a system where kidney donors are paid by the government."

"And kidneys are what, about eighty percent of all organ transplants?"

"That's right."

"It's also true that in Iran there is virtually no waiting list for a kidney."

"I believe that is correct."

"Now, do you know if the paid donors in Iran are all impoverished, that is to say, is their system simply taking advantage of the poor?"

"I don't know," she said.

"I do," Kristine said brightly. "According to a study done by the NIH, in terms of socio-economic background, there are 'no significant differences' in groups of donors and recipients. So the greatly feared exploitation of the poor is not occurring."

"Apparently not," Ms. Putnam said.

Ken Stern roused himself to say, "Relevance, Your Honor?"

"Seems like a fair question," the judge said. "Ms. Black?"

Kristine said, "Well, Your Honor, I was hoping to find an answer to the question of why our entire organ donation system is governed by Gift Law when that system has such an embarrassingly low success rate, especially in light of the fact that we know of at least one other system that works far better and saves so many more lives. But let me try another approach."

Kristine turned to face the witness and said, "Ms. Putnam, what is a 'gift' in the legal sense of the Uniform Anatomical Gift Act?"

"It's a legally binding voluntary transfer of something, in this case, an organ, from a donor to a donee without payment," Ms. Putnam said.

"Voluntary, you say. Do I have a choice about that, I mean is there another box to check on the organ donor registry form that would allow me to donate in exchange for a payment?"

"No, then it wouldn't be a gift."

"So in other words, I don't really have a choice," Kristine said. "If I want someone else to have my organs when the time comes, I have to give them away?"

"By law, yes."

"So it's really something that one is forced to do, rather than something one does *voluntarily*, as you would give a real gift, like the one I gave you." Kristine turned to address the jury. "It's a nice-sounding word though, isn't it? Gift. It makes it sound like one person freely giving something to someone else, but, in this case, they're actually *forced* to 'give' it. Gift Law. Almost makes you wonder if the people who decided to call it that had motives for choosing the word. Gift. Maybe it was chosen for P.R. purposes…"

As Kristine was tightening the noose with her line of questioning, I couldn't help but notice the body language of the jurors. It was clear they didn't like what they were hearing. If I had to guess what they were thinking, it would be that they resented the government forcing people to do something while wrapping the whole enterprise up as a lovely gift and leaving twenty people to die every day.

They didn't seem to like that one bit.

And what can I say about Kristine's use of the gift-wrapped package? Truly inspired. It got the jury's attention and made them curious, so they listened to what she had to say, and when she brought the point home, it landed exactly as she wanted. I hesitate to say it but—she has a gift!

I'm no courtroom handicapper, but I believe Kristine won over most of the jury with that performance. So, brava!

18

We didn't know it at the time, but Ethan Chaney was in the courtroom that morning, sitting quietly in the back for an hour or so. As he later testified at his trial, he was there "doing recon because he wanted good intel for his mission." He slipped out during a recess and went about his plan.

Ethan Chaney continued gathering information outside, making notes on the security situation which was somewhat lax owing to the fact that the mobile homes were spread out over two acres of unfenced parking lot. You had to pass through Security to get inside any of the "courtrooms" but anyone could walk onto the parking lot from any direction. After assessing the situation, Ethan Chaney decided he would come from the south.

And then he went home to prepare.

Two hours later, when the judge announced our lunch recess, I said I was going in search of the tapas truck. Miguel and Rebecca didn't want to deal with the media, so they asked me to bring something back. Javeed and Kristine liked the sound of delivery too, so I set off to get lunch for everyone.

Making my way across the lot, I could see TV crews from several local stations. Some were entertainment reporters hoping to get a word with Rebecca Vaughn, others were more interested in Miguel's supporters and the protestors against his cause.

Curt Kingston was there, feeding material to Lynn Mitchum back in the studio. Lynn told Curt not to bother with any of the pro-organ-donor people since there wasn't much sizzle there, so Curt was looking around for a crackpot who wanted to talk.

He made a beeline to the guy wearing a "We are Q" T-shirt.

"What do you think of Mr. Padilla's case against the State?" Curt asked.

The guy shook his head in disdain. "You mean, the *Deep* State, right?" He had the expression of a man who was disgusted that he was talking to a TV reporter.

"Look if you fake media people took the time to decode Podesta's emails you'd know this already," the guy said. "When they say 'donors' they're not talking about *campaign* donors, OK? It's code. They need the organs for the elites." He glanced around like he was about to spill classified information. "That so-called abandoned Cemex facility in Arizona? That's where they take 'em for harvesting." The guy turned and walked away, glancing back once to say, "Educate yourself!"

"I think you can cut," Curt said to his cameraman as he turned to survey the crowd. "Let's see who else is feeling chatty."

My stomach growling, I walked off in the other direction in search of the tapas truck. There were several food trucks parked on Plummer Street: Hot chicken, tacos, sushi, but no tapas. I ordered five hot chicken sandwiches with fries and drinks and returned to my friends.

***

After lunch the trial resumed with Miguel, still acting as co-counsel, calling Dr. Simmons back to the stand.

"Dr. Simmons, you testified earlier about the things that happen leading up to a heart transplant. You said the O.P.O. acquires the organ from the donor as a 'gift' in accordance with the Uniform Anatomical Gift Act. Do I have that right?"

"Yes, that's correct."

"OK, so the O.P.O. gets the 'gift' from the donor and delivers it to the transplant hospital for… free?"

"No," Dr. Simmons said. "The O.P.O. receives a payment for delivering the heart."

"OK. Let me ask you a question: how much does a heart transplant cost?"

"All in? About a million dollars."

"A million dollars," Miguel said. "And, of that, how much am I charged for the heart itself?"

Ken Stern suddenly looked as if he had smelled a fart. "Objection! To suggest that hospitals would charge a desperate patient for a life-saving organ they obtained for nothing? It's a reprehensible supposition."

Dr. Simmons looked to the judge. "Should I answer?"

"Go ahead," the judge said.

"The hospital will charge you about eighty thousand dollars for that heart."

"Objection overruled."

"OK, so the hospital then buys the heart from the O.P.O…."

"Objection," Ken Stern said limply. "The hospital doesn't 'buy' the heart. The hospital…" He paused to think of a better way to phrase it. "…'pays a fee' to obtain a life-giving organ."

The judge said, "And you think that wording changes the nature of the transaction?"

Ken Stern sighed deeply. "No, Your Honor, not really, but it sounds so much less rapacious."

"Overruled."

"So the O.P.O. gets a 'gift,' hands the 'gift' over for a 'fee' and then charges me eighty thousand bucks for it."

I couldn't stand it any longer. I bolted to my feet and proclaimed, "Your Honor! They're treating that heart like it's a piece of property! I move for summary judgment in our favor!"

"Who on earth are you?" the judge said.

"My apologies, Your Honor," I said. "Leonard Stratten, at your service."

The judge motioned for me to take my seat, which I did, since it appeared she meant business. "Do that again," she said, "and you'll spend the night in jail."

I raised my hand in an apologetic surrender followed by the motion of zipping-my-lips. But I had already made my point with the jury, so mission accomplished.

Miguel continued his questioning. "Dr. Simmons, say a heart is in transit from one hospital to another and it's stolen. Would that be a crime since the heart, like other organs, isn't considered property?"

Ken Stern sounded as if his batteries were running down when he said, "Objection. Hypothetical and beyond his expertise."

Miguel looked to Kristine, who called him over for a conference after which Miguel said he wanted to call a new witness.

"And who is this new witness?" the judge asked.

"Any police officer would do," Miguel said. "Just has to be someone qualified to answer the question."

"Any objections, Mr. Stern?"

Ken Stern shook his head miserably and said, "No, Your Honor."

The bailiff went outside to look for someone from the L.A. County Sheriff's Department. While the door was open we could hear the sounds of supporters in the distance chanting, "Miguel! Miguel!" We turned and looked at one another, smiling. It buoyed our spirits knowing they were out there, rooting for us.

The bailiff returned a minute later with a deputy. This time, when the door opened, we heard a chant of, "Hey! Hey! Ho! Ho! Big Organ Has To Go!"

The deputy was sworn in and Miguel posed the question.

The deputy said, "Yes, it would be armed robbery if done with a weapon, strong arm robbery if done with some force but no weapon, and grand theft if no force was used."

"Can you steal something that isn't property?"

The deputy looked perplexed for a moment, as did the judge. The question was a bit metaphysical. "I don't see how that's legally possible," the deputy said.

"So an organ is something that can be stolen which is yet another characteristic of personal property," Miguel said. "Thank you."

Miguel had no more questions for the deputy and Ken Stern was too depressed about the way things were going to cross examine him.

Kristine took over now and called Dr. Simmons back to the stand.

"Dr. Simmons, in the United States, how many organizations are involved with the acquisition and distribution of organs?"

"Just one," he said.

"Just one? That's not very competitive."

Ken Stern somehow managed what appeared to be some minor outrage for this one. "Objection! There's no need for competition. They're not engaged in commerce."

"It certainly sounds like they're engaged in commerce," Kristine said. "All this money and critical resources changing hands like meat at a butcher's shop yet just one company controlling the whole thing."

"Objection overruled," the judge said.

Ken Stern rubbed at the back of his neck as he whined, "It's not a company, Your Honor, it's a non-profit organization."

Kristine said, "Your Honor, I'm suddenly put in mind of monopolies and the Sherman Antitrust Act. How do we know UNOS isn't in cahoots with the hospitals? What's it called?" She snapped her fingers a couple of time. "Oh, collusion! Restraint of trade also comes to mind!"

"Objection," Ken Stern complained. "How can it be restraint of trade? No one's allowed to sell organs."

Kristine looked to the jury as she said, "Except for hospitals which are selling tickers for eighty thousand bucks a pop."

"Objection overruled."

"Thank you, Your Honor," Kristine said. "Now, Dr. Simmons, will everyone on the waiting list for organs receive one?"

"No they won't."

"And will any of them die as a result of not receiving organs?"

"Yes, about twenty-two each day," Dr. Simmons said.

"And why is that?"

"Because demand for organs far exceeds supply."

"In other words, organs are a scarce resource."

Kristine glanced at her watch. "Your Honor, I have a new line of questioning for this witness but I'm afraid it will go longer than you may want for today, so…"

The judge agreed. She banged her gavel and said, "This court is in recess until tomorrow morning at ten. We will see you all then."

***

As everyone in the room collected their belongings to leave, Rebecca eased over to the window and peeked outside.

Miguel said, "How's it look?"

"I count four or five TV crews ready to pounce," she said. "Plus a pack of paparazzi, some autograph hounds, and a couple dozen protestors."

"OK," Miguel said. "What do you have for me?"

"I kept it simple," Rebecca said. She picked up her large canvas tote bag and set it on the plaintiff's table. She unsnapped it and said, "Catholic priest or gangbanger?"

Miguel stared at her in disbelief before he said, "Really…"

"What were you expecting, pirate?"

"How about stockbroker or lawyer?"

"That's what you look like now," Rebecca said. "In fact if I was trying to disguise a priest, a pirate, or a gang member, I'd put 'em in your current outfit."

"Fine," Miguel said, slipping off his suit coat. "Stereotypes notwithstanding, I think I'd rather be seen as a gang member than a Catholic priest."

"Understandable," Rebecca said.

Javeed said, "Didn't you just stereotype priests?"

Rebecca pulled a blue do-rag and a black horseshoe mustache from her bag. She handed those to Miguel and said, "Start with that."

Rebecca slipped a long blonde wig over her famous brunette bob and topped it with a floppy sun hat.

"How do I make the mustache stick?"

Rebecca looked at me. "Leonard, could you handle that? There's spirit gum in the bag."

I found the glue and got to work on the mustache. I had never been this close to Miguel. He was a bit ashy but I didn't think this was the time or place to bring that up, so I made a note to myself to buy some quality moisturizer as a gift.

While I worked on the mustache, Rebecca put a beauty mark on her right cheek and clipped on a large nose ring and a pair of black framed cat-eye glasses. Then she stepped into a pair of maroon leggings and out of her skirt which she stuffed into the bag.

The mustache and do-rag in place, Rebecca and Kristine stepped back to look Miguel over.

"The shirt's all wrong," Kristine said, shaking her head.

Rebecca agreed. She rooted through her bag until she found a blue denim shirt with the sleeves torn off. "Try this."

Miguel swapped his button-down white oxford for the sleeveless denim.

"That works." Rebecca and Kristine nodded their approval.

"OK," Rebecca said to Miguel. "Walk out like you're on your phone and keep it on the crowd side of your face." She looked at everyone and said, "Let's go."

Miguel and Rebecca fell in behind a couple of the jurors as they walked out of the trailer. Kristine, Javeed, and I walked out a moment later. One of the paparazzi yelled, "Is Rebecca Vaughn in there?"

"Yes, she was right behind us," I said, pointing back at the door. "I believe she'll be out in just a moment." We kept walking.

The same guy in the crowd then called out, "Hey! Aren't you the guy who shot that man in Santa Monica two nights ago?"

Rebecca and Miguel stopped and turned to look back in surprise. Kristine and Javeed took a step away from me and stared as I said, "What?" I forced a laugh. "No, you've obviously got me confused with someone else." I kept walking.

"You're dressed just like him!"

"No crime in being fashionable," I said, still on the move.

"Is that the cane gun you shot him with?" the man asked.

You could hear the cameras snapping like firecrackers but at least no one was looking for Miguel or Rebecca Vaughn any more.

"Cane gun?" I glanced down at my cane but made sure not to hold it up for photographs. "No, I'm sorry, this is just a walking stick." I looked back to the trailer door and pointed. "Oh, there's Ms. Vaughn now!"

Fortunately they fell for it and went chasing after some poor woman who was walking off in the other direction, allowing us to escape.

We took our separate cars and met back at ICU as we had planned.

***

I was last to arrive. The others were at a table in the back. Naturally they had taken the time to search for news stories about the shooting. I knew they'd want some answers.

"It was self-defense," I said. "The man was trying to rob me at gunpoint. I did what I had to do."

"That's so scary," Rebecca said, reaching over to touch my hand. "But the cane gun is very cool! So James Bond!"

"Quick question," Javeed said. "Did it just slip your mind that you shot a man two nights ago? I mean, did you simply forget to tell us?"

"Honestly, I didn't want anyone to know," I said. "I wanted to keep it as quiet as possible lest it interfere with our project. I had no way of knowing, for example, if Ms. Vaughn might bow out because she didn't want to be associated with what happened. Or if her representatives might have a problem with it. So I kept quiet."

"Are you kidding?" Rebecca said. "My agent was beside herself when I told her what happened. I think CIA wants to rep you now!"

"Well, there's a silver lining—"

"Wait a second," Miguel said, stabbing a finger at his phone screen. "The guy who tried to rob you? Says here his name is McElheny. Isn't that the guy you said conned you out of fifty thousand bucks back in New York?"

"What? No, that was a chap by the name of McNamara," I said, surprised that Miguel had remembered the name. "By the way, does it say how the man's doing? I don't feel bad about shooting the chap, but I'd rather not have his death on my conscience." In truth, I knew I would manage just fine either way but thought this sounded better.

Kristine's phone chimed a text just as Miguel said, "It says he's critical but stable."

"Well, that's a relief."

Miguel gazed into the middle distance looking somewhat mystified as he said, "I could have sworn it was McElheny…"

Looking for a distraction, I focused on Kristine's shocked reaction to the text she had received. I said, "Kristine? Everything alright?"

"You're not going to believe this," she said. "Someone did it."

"Did what?" I said. "What are you looking at?"

"A newspaper article a friend of mine sent, a lawyer," Kristine said. "I told him about Miguel's case."

"And?"

Kristine read from the article, "Sixty-three-year-old Winston Tremblay, diagnosed with ALS, was allowed to donate his organs following a medically assisted death."

Miguel said, "What? When? Where?"

"I'm still reading…" Kristine said. "Uhhh, it was last year."

"So that's good for us, right?" Miguel said. "Legal precedent?"

She read from the article: "It came after a decision from the Superior Court of... damn," Kristine said.

"What?"

"No help," she said.

"Why not?"

"This was in Canada."

"Canada?"

"Yeah, you know, moose, hockey, poutine..."

"And national health care," Javeed said.

"So that doesn't help at all?"

"Afraid not," Kristine said. "Canadian judicial rulings have no bearing in U.S. courts."

"What if I moved there?"

"Wouldn't help," Kristine said. "You have to live there for a few years before you can become a citizen."

"What if I moved there and stole someone's identity?"

"Probably easier to find someone from a Chinese firing squad," Javeed said.

"About all we can do is tell the jury in closing arguments that our friends to the north thought it over and approved of the idea," Kristine said.

"Aren't Canadians famous for being polite? Maybe they'd just be nice and take my organs..."

***

I was astonished by the size of the crowd. It must have been ten times the size of the day before. I can't speak for the others, but I had to park four blocks away.

One of the reasons for the crowd was that Creative International Agency had put their entire social media department to work pumping up our project. Now that Ace Studios was at least nominally committed, they wanted to do all they could to increase brand awareness for *The Organ Grinders*!

They never mentioned that the trial was under way, but some hardcore Rebecca Vaughn fans knew about it, posted the information, and it went viral. Everyone who was following #organguy! and #cultureofdeath! knew about it.

As a side note you should know I felt like a fool that day as I walked toward the court and, I fear, I looked like one as well. You see, in an effort to throw off the paparazzi, for the first time since my childhood I was wearing a baseball cap. A blue Dodgers cap. It didn't match anything I was wearing, not my tie, not my shirt, not even my pocket square. But if they were looking for someone wearing a fedora, they would look past me. I'm sure I looked ridiculous, but it was a price I was willing to pay if it meant I could slip past the jackals of the press unnoticed.

I was also carrying a different, non-lethal, walking stick. On the chance that someone challenged me about it, I could "prove" it was just a cane and I wasn't the man they were looking for.

Ahead of me I saw people getting out of a minivan. A man with two children. The man pulled something from the back and put it on one of kids. It was an old-fashioned sandwich board saying: *My mom needs a kidney. O-positive. 888-222-2222. Please help.* The man put one on the other child and then donned a larger one with the same message, substituting "wife" for "mom."

There were others looking for hope as well. Some wore T-shirts with their plea printed on them, others were handing out flyers.

The closer I got, the more signs I came into view.

Over here: I Support #organguy!

Over there: #cultureofdeath! Is Here!

Across the street: My Body, My Property!

Up ahead: Don't Tread On My Organs!

In the distance: TAPAS!

Where was this elusive food truck? I wondered.

The different factions were milling about. Those in favor of assisted death were gathering to the east, those opposed were on the north intermingling with a nasty-looking bunch of anti-organ-donor protestors. Some were there in favor of everything. Some were against it all. Some were getting their groups organized, others were quietly working social media.

The Sheriff's Department, charged with security for the court system, had brought in a few more deputies to keep control, but it was hardly an overwhelming police force. They clearly underestimated the turnout.

Ethan Chaney was watching it all from his car as he prepared himself.

19

Once the trial resumed, Kristine had Miguel take over to question the next witness. He reminded the jury of the testimony from Dr. Simmons. "He told us that the demand for organs exceeds supply. In other words, organs are a scarce commodity," he said. "So, keeping that word—scarce—in mind, I would like to call to the stand Professor James Fowler."

Once sworn in, Professor Fowler listed his bona fides as a recognized expert in the areas of Economics and Property Law. Indeed he spoke as if quoting lines from the textbook he wrote.

"Professor Fowler," Miguel said. "Why do we have property rights?"

"Their fundamental purpose," he said, "is the elimination of destructive competition for control of economic resources."

"Well," Miguel said, "property rights don't eliminate destructive competition so much as they provide a remedy for when it happens, right? It's not as though the existence of property rights brought an end to property crimes."

"Fair enough," the professor said. "Well-defined and enforced property rights are designed to discourage competition by violence and to encourage competition by peaceful means. And, as you say, they provide a remedy for when violations do occur."

"Right, so yesterday Dr. Simmons made the point that organs are a scarce resource," Miguel said. "Can you tell us, Professor, does the concept of scarcity play a role in the philosophy of property rights?"

"Yes. It's one of the foundational ideas."

Hello, dear reader, it's me again. Sorry to interrupt, but, trust me, it's in your best interest. At this point Miguel and Professor Fowler went down a long and tiresome road during which they explored the political philosophies of John Locke and David Hume including extensive digressions on Chapter V of Locke's *Second Treatise of Government: Of Property*. And Hume's *Treatise of Human Nature*. Fascinating stuff, if Professor Fowler is to be believed but, so far as I know, neither has had their work turned into a movie starring Oprah Winfrey which I believe is evidence to the contrary.

In any event, as they subjected the jury to this torture, some of us in the gallery couldn't help but notice the clamor from the gathering crowd of protestors. Distant cries of "Organ Guy! Organ Guy!" echoed down the shallow canyons between the mobile homes, followed by equally passionate voices calling out with "Culture of Death! Culture of Death!" I got the sense things were too volatile out there for me to consider going in search of the mysterious tapas food truck.

Meanwhile Professor Fowler was saying, "Once a resource becomes scarce, those who desire the resource will struggle to control it. This leads to conflict where the more powerful party dispossesses the weaker party of the resource. This instability of possession is the chief impediment to society and thus something the law tries to prevent by investing the party in possession of the scarce resource with a property right."

Miguel said, "The ultimate finding in Moore v. Regents was that Mr. Moore's blood and tissue and subparts were his own personal property and thus he had a right to share in profits derived from same. Do I have that right?"

"That's correct," the professor said.

"So in this country we have agreed that blood, sperm, eggs, and bone marrow, among other things, are property."

"Yes."

"Would you say that any of those things are scarce?"

"Not in the common usage of the word, but you have to understand, in economic terminology, the word 'scarce' just means that the demand for a resource exceeds the supply of the resource. Take cars, for example," the professor said. "There are millions of cars out there, so they're not scarce in the common use of the word. But there are more people who want cars than can acquire them."

"So if blood is considered scarce enough to warrant being given the protection of property rights, wouldn't you think kidneys should be afforded the same protection?"

"That's not up to me," the professor said. "But I would think so."

Miguel pointed at the witness. "A moment ago you said property rights are bestowed in order to prevent a stronger party from dispossessing a weaker party from their property."

"That's correct."

"Which would you say is the stronger party of the following two: an individual citizen or a Federally mandated organization like UNOS?"

"UNOS is clearly the stronger party."

"And yet through the disingenuous use of Gift Law, they are allowed to dispossess individual citizens of their organs."

Ken Stern arose, as if awakened from a long sleep, and said, "Objection, Your Honor, what's the question?"

"Yes," the judge said. "What's your point?"

Miguel replied, "Your Honor, the point is my parts are my property and I should be allowed to do with my property as I wish so long as I don't impinge upon the rights of anyone else."

I noticed a few members of the jury casting nervous glances toward the windows on the side of the trailer where the boisterous crowds were protesting.

"Very good, Mr. Padilla," the judge said. "Now, Mr. Stern, would you like to make any points to the contrary?

"Yes, Your Honor," he said. "If I might cite Justice Arabian from his opinion in Moore v. Regents: 'I am concerned about the conflicting moral values at stake and the profound implications of recognizing a property interest in body parts. The ramifications of this are greatly feared.'"

Miguel looked at the jury and said, "Greatly feared by whom? Certainly not by those who might benefit from it. Or their families or their friends for that matter."

"I believe Justice Arabian was making a broader point about the instinctive revulsion at denial of bodily integrity," Ken Stern said like a man who wasn't buying the very thing he was selling.

The judge said, "What does that even mean?"

"I don't know, Your Honor," Ken Stern said. "It's something I read somewhere. But if it pleases the court I do have an amicus brief I would like to present."

"And who is this friend of the court?"

Ken Stern gestured toward the noisy crowd and said, "It's one of the groups protesting out there." He glanced at his notes. "An organization calling themselves Theocrats Against Physician Assisted Suicide."

The judge thought about it for a second. "Theocrats Against Physician Assisted Suicide? T.A.P.A.S. TAPAS? The acronym for their organization means Spanish appetizers? I saw that sign outside," the judge said. "I thought it was advertising for a food truck."

"I don't understand the connection either, Your Honor," Ken Stern said. "Still, they asked to be heard."

"Very well," the judge said. "Proceed."

"They're objecting on religious grounds," Mr. Stern said. "They say their religious liberty is under attack.

The judge mumbled, "Color me shocked."

Ken Stern read the prepared statement. "We, the Theocrats Against Physician Assisted Suicide have a deeply held religious belief that Mr. Padilla should embrace the slow and painful death our Lord has seen in His wisdom to give unto him. As the sainted Mother Teresa said,

'There is something beautiful in seeing the sick and poor accept their lot, to suffer it like Christ's Passion. The world gains much from their suffering.'"

"I object!" Kristine said. "This organization lacks standing in the matter."

"That's not all they're lacking," the judge said. "Objection sustained."

"Your Honor, I'm curious," Miguel said. "What is the State's interest in denying my request?"

"I haven't the foggiest, Mr. Padilla," the judge said. "Perhaps they just want to keep you alive so you're paying taxes. Now, Mr. Stern, do you have anything further to say?"

He hung his head and said, "Nothing worthwhile, Your Honor."

***

We all noticed the crowd outside had grown steadily larger and—from the sounds of it—more agitated, all day. We could hear the opposing camps as they tried to shout each other down. "Organ Guy!" followed by "Culture of Death!" over and over.

Now and then we could hear someone from the Sheriff's Department on a bullhorn directing people to move back or to keep it civil.

Ethan Chaney was out there, snaking through the crowd. At one point he picked up a discarded protest sign that was taped to a metal pipe so he would blend in better.

Around this time someone posted the wrong trailer number on social media. One faction after another started moving in that direction until there was a large group protesting outside what turned out to be a Small Claims Court trial involving a woman suing her ex-boyfriend for $52.77 after he moved out and took her entire supply of cherry-flavored edible underwear with him.

But Ethan Chaney knew where Miguel's trial was and he started redirecting the protestors in that direction. He hoisted his sign and yelled, "It's this way!"

As the disturbance grew, the judge noticed some of the people in the gallery looking around nervously and whispering about the crowd outside.

The judge banged her gavel. "Order! Quiet!" She waited until she had everyone's attention.

"That's better," the judge said. "Now, to the detriment of many, the law changes slowly. Laws on organ donation written decades ago are woefully outdated. In the absence of new laws, those in possession of human tissue—which is to say all of us—will be vulnerable to being dispossessed of our property by a stronger party."

The protestors were heading toward our trailer, their chants growing louder as they approached. Ethan Chaney fell back into the roil and churn of the crowd as he separated the sign from the pipe.

The judge continued: "This is contrary to the law's aim of protecting peaceful possession. And the best way to do that is to allocate property rights in these scarce resources, and in time I suspect this will happen. In fact what happens today may be a part of that change. Now, Mr. Padilla, before I instruct the jury and they go to deliberate, do you wish to make a final statement to the court?"

"Yes, thank you, Your Honor," he said.

A voice on a bullhorn announced something, but it was indistinct inside our trailer. The agitated crowd jeered the announcement whatever it was. Everyone in the court glanced out the windows before returning their attention to the proceedings.

Miguel gestured at the unseen crowd and said, "These protesters are aghast at the notion of the body as property in the same way others were aghast at the very notion of transplants in 1968." Miguel looked at the jury. "Fifty years ago the public response to the first organ transplant was vicious, primitive, and superstitious. The doctors were vilified for playing God, for doing the unnatural. They were threatened personally and professionally by those who feared progress. Now? Transplants are as controversial as an appendectomy."

The chants grew louder. "Organ Guy! Organ Guy!"

The jury members looked at one another nervously as Miguel gestured at the unseen rabble.

"Progress is always met with hostility," Miguel said. "It doesn't matter if you're promoting civil rights or advances in medical treatment, the members of the Flat Earth Society will demand that you turn back. And when they demand that, you know it's time to go forward. Your Honor, members of the jury, I'm just trying to do some good before I'm gone. I simply want to be allowed to exercise my rights and help save some lives. I don't think I'm asking too much," Miguel said.

The judge let that sink in before she said, "Thank you, Mr. Padilla. I wish you luck." She turned to the jury. "Now, before I give instructions—"

Our frayed nerves snapped when that pipe shattered the window, spraying shards of glass into the courtroom. A few people screamed.

Ethan Chaney then tossed something through the broken window. It hit the floor and rolled unevenly toward Miguel.

It happened so fast. And it was horrible.

Miguel shoved Kristine away, yelling, "Get down!"

Kristine, falling backwards, seeing what was going to happen, pleading, "Don't!"

Miguel threw himself on top of it.

***

The blast killed Miguel instantly. But he saved our lives.

Miguel's body redirected much of the energy through the floor of the cheaply made trailer. The undersized joists topped with cheap particle board and thin laminate gave way to the explosion sending most of the shrapnel down into the asphalt below.

The sound of the detonation brought an immediate police response. Dozens of sheriff's deputies and LAPD officers who were in the area descended on our trailer. The protestors were moved back to the edge of the parking lot, corralled and had their statements taken.

The bomb squad and the FBI were there within seven minutes.

Ethan Chaney tried to run, but he was held by some of Miguel's supporters until a deputy took him away in cuffs. As they shoved him into the back of the cruiser he was yelling incoherently about how he was saving everyone from the culture of death.

We were all in shock. Kristine and Javeed held each other, crying uncontrollably. Rebecca Vaughn and I were too stunned to feel the sorrow yet. We hugged one another and didn't let go. We were still shaking as the police led us all out of the trailer.

There was nothing the medics could do for Miguel. His body remained where it was for a time as crime scene investigators gathered their information.

At his trial we learned that Ethan Chaney had spent time in a chat room on the dark web, a meeting place where he knew a lot of EOD vets hung out. He told them he was going to take an old car out to the desert and blow it up for fun and was soliciting ideas on everyone's favorite and cheapest IED made with household chemicals.

One guy who remembered Ethan told him to forget about making an IED. Instead he suggested Ethan go to a particular booth at a gun show out in the Inland Empire. "Tell him Rusty sent you," the guy said. "He'll fix you up with something fun."

Sure enough the man sold Ethan Chaney a couple of M-67 fragmentation grenades for two hundred dollars. Stolen army surplus, tons of them around. Ethan still had one in his pocket when he was arrested.

***

There was talk of having a large public memorial for Miguel, but we realized the TAPAS people and others would likely stage a protest and take the focus off the celebration of our friend's life and his sacrifice.

So when the day came, it was just the four of us and Miguel's ashes. We went to Griffith Park late that afternoon and sat around a table at one of the picnic areas. We poured large glasses of tangeritas and shared stories about Miguel.

Kristine said a beautiful and uplifting prayer about the blessings that Miguel had brought into our lives.

Rebecca Vaughn sang a Leonard Cohen song that brought tears to our eyes.

Miguel hadn't specified where he wanted his ashes spread, so we discussed some options and took a vote. After finishing the second jug of tangeritas, we snuck into Dodger Stadium and spread Miguel's ashes all over the playing field amid a great deal of drunken giggling.

When the ashes were all dispersed, we stood at second base and looked around. "Miguel wanted to do something of great consequence before he died," I said. "And he did it. We are blessed to have known him."

***

Sad as I was that Miguel was gone, at least now I knew how the story ended.

The question was how would I write it for the stage?

The first draft ended with the glass breaking, the grenade landing at Miguel's feet and him jumping on it. Blackout. Then a blinding flash of light and a boom!

The End.

It was theatrical and abrupt and I liked that. Just stun the audience and send them home, shocked that it happened that way.

But perhaps it was too abrupt.

So I went back to the drawing board and took another shot at it.

After the window is shattered and the grenade lands at Miguel's feet...

(The lights go out except for a spot on Miguel who stares at the grenade.)

MIGUEL	You've got to be kidding. That's a terrible idea.

(LEONARD *joins* MIGUEL *in the spotlight, putting his arm over* MIGUEL's *shoulder*)

LEONARD	No, no, no, it's perfect! We couldn't ask for a better ending!
MIGUEL	You realize I've got to jump on that, right? Plus it's so… obvious.
LEONARD	No, think of it as… unambiguous.

(KRISTINE *joins them in the spotlight*)

KRISTINE	God bless you, Miguel.

(JAVEED *joins them*)

JAVEED	You have alternatives!
LEONARD	Don't listen to him, Miguel. You have to do this. If you don't, it ruins the ending.
MIGUEL	But I want to know the verdict.
LEONARD	No, it plays better this way. Let them think about it. Give them something to talk about on the way home.
MIGUEL	If you say so. Now, just promise you'll tell my story.

LEONARD	You have my word.
MIGUEL	Then I guess that's it. Well, guys, it's been fun. Whaddya say, once more for the road?

(MIGUEL *thrusts a hand in the air as if holding a rapier*)

MIGUEL	Lex!

(KRISTINE *joins him*)

KRISTINE	Clavatoris!

(JAVEED *joins them*)

JAVEED	Designati!

(LEONARD *joins, using his cane as rapier*)

LEONARD	Rescindenda!
EVERYBODY	Est!

(*Blackout followed by A BLINDING FLASH and an EXPLOSION! There is a pause before lights slowly come up to dim*)

Silence as everyone stares, stunned at what has happened. MIGUEL lies on the floor, face down.
The TV screens all come back on and all the faces look down to where MIGUEL lies. Then they all close their eyes and the screens go black. After a moment, one of the TV screens flickers back to life. It's LYNN MITCHUM, doing a stand-up.

LYNN MITCHUM   In a remarkable exhibition of altruism,
a man died in a California courtroom
today after throwing himself onto a live
grenade, likely saving the lives of thirty
others. Miguel Padilla was said to have
had a monumental hero complex in
addition to a subconscious desire for
fame. Otherwise, he was a simple man
who wanted nothing more out of life
than to help others and bring an end to
the designated hitter rule.

(The TV screen goes black as does the stage)

*In the darkness, over what will doubtlessly be thunderous applause
from our audience, the cast begins to HUM the melody of "God Rest Ye
Merry Gentlemen."
After a bar or two of humming to get the audience's attention,
the lights come up.
The courtroom is gone. It has been replaced by a row of reclining chairs
and an equal number of hemodialysis machines.
The characters are seated in the chairs and connected to machines.
It is a dialysis clinic.
From above, a large, garish banner unfurls, like a sideshow freak sign:*

THE ORGAN GRINDERS!
by
Leonard Stratten

(The cast sings to the established tune)

MIGUEL   You need a nice pink pancreas,
My surgeon said to me.

KRISTINE

The one you've got is all but shot,
On this we all agree.

JAVEED

Get on the list and do it now,
Or you'll be history…

EVERYBODY

And lots of discomfort and oy,
Discomfort and oy,
And lots of discomfort, oy vey.

MIGUEL

What does it do,
I have no clue,
But without you won't thrive.

KEN STERN

It has to do with insulin,
You need to be alive.

THE JUDGE

The wait's too long,
The part's been used,
Of life you'll be deprived.

EVERYBODY

And lots of discomfort and oy,
Discomfort and oy,
And lots of discomfort, oy vey!

Epilogue

SOME MONTHS LATER

I'm pleased to report that *The Organ Grinders!* opened to uniformly glowing reviews at the August Playhouse. Rebecca Vaughn would go on to win an Ovation Award for her performance. It was the hardest ticket in town for months.

The after-party of the premier was held in the theater's opulent lobby, a stunning hall done in the French baroque style with glorious crystal chandeliers dropping thirty-five feet from the ceiling, magnificent red velvet drapery caressing the walls, and gold leaf on every inch of the spectacular rococo molding. It looked like a fairytale palace.

Kristine, Javeed, and I stood near the top of one of the sweeping staircases, taking in the glorious scene below as stars of the stage and screen mingled with the power brokers of the entertainment industry. Kristine and Javeed were dressed to the nines, as they say. No surprise to anyone that I was dressed to ten.

At one point Kristine slipped her arm around my waist, pulled me closer, and said, "I'm so glad you showed up."

"To the premier of my own show? What did you expect?"

"No, in Miguel's life," she said. "In *our* lives."

It made me smile. "If memory serves, that wasn't your initial reaction," I chided.

"Oh, give her a break," Javeed said. "How could she have known all this was coming?"

I turned and looked at Javeed as you would a guilty child. "Listen to you," I said. "How did you describe it? *Les Miz* on the cheap but with Miguel's organs instead of French peasants?"

"Yeah, well…"

Kristine leaned in to add, "He also said it wasn't something with the grandeur of opera so much as a collection of songs you'd stolen."

"Yes, that's true," I said. "But, in Javeed's defense, I should point out he was prompted by your accusation of copyright infringement."

She laughed and said, "I'm a lawyer, I can't help it."

"And, by the way, thanks for the help on that bit of Cole Porter."

"Don't mention it," Kristine said.

"Perhaps you should consider adding intellectual property rights to your legal repertoire."

"Well, I might," she said slyly, "but only in cases that relate to Constitutional Law."

Javeed and I looked at her for further elucidation.

"I got an offer from a big firm today," Kristine said. "They were impressed by the originality of my arguments in Miguel's case."

"So it's goodbye Wills and Trusts?"

"If I never have to explain probate to another person it will be too soon," she said. "Also, I think Miguel was right that I should get out of my comfort zone and stretch a bit." She touched her hand over heart then pointed subtly at the heavens where she knew Miguel was watching.

I kissed her cheek and said, "Congratulations!"

"You'll be a star," Javeed said. "And Miguel would be so proud and happy for you."

In the crowd below I noticed Rebecca Vaughn chatting casually with one of her co-stars when her face suddenly lit up at the sight of an approaching gentleman. She broke from her chat and gave the man a warm, lingering hug.

I nudged Javeed and said, "Who is that with Rebecca?"

He looked. "Oh, that's Mr. Kaye," he said.

It took me a moment to remember. "The man who introduced us to Dr. Brewer? The one you met at that… hospital?"

"That's him."

It made me wonder but I never asked how she knew him. It was none of my business.

"Well, if you two don't mind," Javeed said, nodding toward the crowd below, "I'm going to go have a word with Ms. Vaughn."

"Ahh." I elbowed Kristine. "I believe the boy is smitten."

"Hang on," Kristine said. "I'm coming with you."

"You fancy Ms. Vaughn too?"

"What? No," she said. "I thought I'd introduce myself to Mr. Kaye, give him my number. Seems like the type who might need an attorney some day."

As I watched the two of them glide down the stairs, I caught a slight commotion out of the corner of my eye.

It was a man at the door, agitated and trying to push his way past Security, as sometimes happens at events such as this.

I couldn't get a good look at his face, so, being cautious, I adjusted the hand on my cane and flicked the safety off with my thumb. Just in case it was McElheny.

Also Available

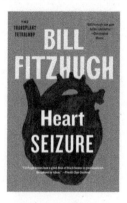

Heart Seizure
(The Transplant Tetralogy, Book 1)

Spence Tailor, a lawyer with an actual set of principals, loves his mama, Rose.

Rose – with advanced cardiomyopathy and a rare blood type – is scheduled for a heart transplant. But when the president's heart craps out during a photo op three months before the national election, the White House chief of staff orders the FBI to seize the heart that was going to Rose – all in the name of democracy.

But Spence isn't about to let anybody steal what rightfully belongs to his mom. So with the help of his reluctant older brother, they hijack the heart, inadvertently kidnap a beautiful cardiac surgery resident, and take to the road in a '65 Mustang – with all the president's men in potentially murderous pursuit.

OUT NOW

Also Available

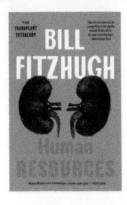

Human Resources
(The Transplant Tetralogy, Book 2)

Jake Trapper isn't your average organ acquisition specialist. He's the best in L.A. But Jake has a soft spot for underdogs and his current case is Angel, a young girl from a broken home. She needs a kidney. So Jake makes a deal with a broker and gets seduced into the kidney business.

When a potential organ donor is killed, Jake meets LAPD Homicide Detective Megan Densmore who enlists Jake to help with the investigation. Enter Special Agent Fuller, a Fed looking into the black market angle. He's an oddball with an architecture fetish and an endless supply of strange tales to tell.

As more bodies surface, Special Agent Fuller turns a suspicious eye toward Jake and the noose tightens, threatening to reveal Jake's dirty little secret.

Human Resources is a darkly comic thriller with heart, and lungs, and kidneys… and a botched monkey kidnapping.

COMING SOON

About the Transplant Tetralogy

Four different tales that consider the possibilities, bizarre inevitabilities, and unintended consequences of one of the greatest achievements of medical science. Each instalment of the Transplant Tetralogy takes you on a darkly comic exploration of the world of organ transplants. This is what happens when demand exceeds supply…

Further titles in the Transplant Tetralogy:

Heart Seizure
Human Resources
The Organ Grinders
A Perfect Harvest

Other series by Bill Fitzhugh:

ASSASSIN BUGS
Pest Control
The Exterminators

DJ RICK SHANNON
Radio Activity
Highway 61 Resurfaced

OTHER
Cross Dressing
Fender Benders

About the Author

Bill Fitzhugh is the author of eleven novels. He still has all of his original organs and plans to keep it that way until the very end, at which point he is willing to let the doctors divvy them up among anyone (with the exception of politicians) who might need them. However, he makes no promises about the quality of his liver. He lives in Los Angeles with his wife and all of her organs.

Note from the Publisher

If you enjoyed this book, we are delighted to share also
The Bug Job, a new short story by Bill Fitzhugh.
To get your **free copy of The Bug Job**, as well as receive
news of further releases by Bill Fitzhugh, sign up at http://
farragobooks.com/billfitzhugh-signup